W9-AWA-370

ALTERING FATE

OTHER BOOKS FROM MICHAEL LEWIS

The Origins of Intelligence: Infancy and Early Childhood
(New York: Plenum, 1976)

Social Cognition and the Acquisition of Self
(with J. Brooks-Gunn) (New York: Plenum, 1979)

Children's Emotions and Moods
(with L. Michalson) (New York: Plenum, 1983)

Beyond the Dyad
(New York: Plenum, 1984)

Learning Disabilities and Prenatal Risk
(Champaign: University of Illinois Press, 1986)

Shame: The Exposed Self
(New York: Free Press, 1992; pbk., 1995)

Handbook of Emotions
(with Jeannette M. Haviland) (New York: Guilford, 1993)

Lying and Deception in Everyday Life
(with Carolyn Saarni) (New York: Guilford, 1993)

ALTERING FATE

*Why the Past
Does Not Predict
the Future*

MICHAEL LEWIS

THE GUILFORD PRESS
New York London

© 1997 Michael Lewis
Published by The Guilford Press
A Division of Guilford Publications, Inc.
72 Spring Street, New York, NY 10012

All rights reserved

No part of this book may be reproduced, stored in a retrieval
system, or transmitted, in any form or by any means, electronic,
mechanical, photocopying, microfilming, recording, or otherwise,
without written permission from the Publisher.

Printed in the United States of America

This book is printed on acid-free paper.

Last digit is print number: 9 8 7 6 5 4 3 2 1

Library of Congress Cataloging-in-Publication Data

Lewis, Michael, 1937 Jan. 10–
   Altering fate : why the past does not predict the future /
Michael Lewis.
     p. cm.
   Includes bibliographical references and index.
   ISBN 0-89862-856-3 (hard)
   1. Context effects (Psychology) 2. Developmental
psychology—Philosophy. 3. Determinism
(Philosophy)—Controversial literature. I. Title.
BF714.L48   1997
155—dc21   96-52568
                                    CIP

For the men of my life, debts I gladly acknowledge:

To Ben, my father, who taught me how to love by giving.
To Morris, my uncle, who taught me about books and melons.
To Benjamin, my son, who teaches me still about other
   ways of being.

in my own life moments that were anything but orderly. How then could I believe in an orderly and predictable life course and at the same time view my own life as punctuated by the unknown and unpredictable? The fact was that I did. I think I have been able to live with both views because I needed to believe in spite of what I had witnessed. My need for identity, that it be "me" across time and place, required that I construct a narrative, a story of me. This need for a personal story led me and leads me still to construct a beginning and a middle and to imagine an end—a progression.

This need in me, I believe, is a common need, one that I share with others. We all need our sense of ourselves; the idea of "me" is powerful and needs to be preserved. Identity requires a story, and the best story we have, in spite of what may actually happen, is the story of progress, continuity, gradualism, and orderliness.

I have written this book to confront these two very different views of human development. In it I will argue that accidents and chance encounters are part of life. That life is not orderly or predictable and thus the past does not seal our fate. Instead, I will argue for a view of life as complex and emerging, where the task is always adaptation to the present.

Because our understanding of how humans develop bears on how we parent and how the society tries to affect lives of children and families, our view of development must impact on social policy. This book therefore not only confronts the topic of development but also addresses how social policy and parenting are affected by our beliefs. My argument is no dry comment on some academic discussion but rather draws us into our daily life with our children and ourselves.

This book is based mainly on the study of development during infancy and early childhood. This focus is no accident. To begin with, it is the content area that I have spent much of my life exploring and therefore know best. Besides, the modern study of development was and remains largely the study of infancy and early childhood. That is both its strength and its weakness—strength because it has allowed us to build up a sizable body of information on one area of development, weakness since it has neglected other periods in the life cycle. The study of these other periods of life could reveal that the conclusions reached from the study of early childhood are too harsh: that there is order and regularity and that the organismic model, as we often define development, can be observed and studied. While this may be the case, I do not think it is so.

The students and colleagues I have worked with over the years have

PREFACE

M y life has been made up of a series of accidents and chance encounters. I was the second child to a family of immigrants. Left-handed and dyslexic, throughout school I followed my sister, who was exceptionally talented, while I just managed to pass. I could not read well and was hit for using my left hand to write. Suddenly the people around me started to sicken and die. First, when I was six years old, my grandmother, who lived with us. Then my mother died when I was eight, and my favorite uncle when I was thirteen. By the time I was eighteen my favorite aunt had moved away and my father had died.

Suddenly I was without family and home, where once I had had no concern. I left for the Moore School of Electrical Engineering at the University of Pennsylvania, where I majored in engineering because of my lack of language skills. After two years—and hearing a lecture by a well-known sociologist—I switched to demography. Graduating without any idea of what to do next, I worked for a year before starting graduate school in clinical psychology. While in my first year, I became interested in physiological psychology and then in problems in development. Because my professor knew of a job opening at Fels Research Institute in Ohio, I went off to the interview and found myself married and living on a pig farm in southeastern Ohio.

These are the fragments of a life well lived, a life full of accidents and chance encounters. As I review my life, it appears more like a trail of turns and twists than an orderly progression. Yet I have spent the last thirty-five years trying to understand how humans develop, as if there were some predictability. At the same time that I was searching for the orderliness in the lives of others, I was experiencing and had experienced greatly aided my studies. I wish I could acknowledge each of them in some more explicit fashion, for I have learned much from each of them, as I hope they have from me. Over the last thirty years there have been many, and it is a source of pride to me to have had the opportunity to teach and work with so many of the leaders in the field of development. I mention many of them now and in the references found in the following chapters.

My deep appreciation to Heidi Als, Steven Alessandri, Margaret Bendersky, Richard Brinker, Linda Michalson Brinker, Jeanne Brooks Gunn, Deborah Coates, Peggy Ban De Wolfe, Rose Di Biase, Carol Pope Edwards, Saul Feinman, Candice Feiring, Nathan Fox, Roy Freedle, Susan Goldberg, Jeannette Haviland, John Jaskir, Barbara Louis, Harry McGurk, Stuart Miller, Douglas Ramsay, Saul Rosenthal, Carolyn Saarni, Catherine Stanger, Margaret Sullivan, Gail Wasserman, Aileen Wehren, Marsha Weinraub, Louise Cherry Wilkinson, John Worobey, and Jerry Young.

As always, my many thanks and deep appreciation to Ruth Gitlen, whose fine eye and typing skills helped bring the manuscript into existence. Many thanks to Cynthia Hall and Jennifer Cole, who also helped with the typing, and to Despina Laverick and Stacey Napoli for helping with the references. Barbara Louis's skills at proofreading, as well as her helpful comments, made the manuscript more readable. Lawrence A. Pervin and Leonard Rosenblum, my dearest friends and colleagues, read an earlier draft, as did my son, Benjamin. I thank them for their suggestions and criticisms, which certainly have made the content clearer, if not more valid. Richard M. Lerner and Hayne W. Reese, longtime contextualists, educated me about nuances that I had missed. The book, I hope, is much improved by their helpful comments. Finally, to Chris Benton, my editor, I owe a debt herein recognized. She not only enhanced this work's readability but led me to make sure that what it says makes sense to anyone who reads it.

I am particularly indebted to the Robert Wood Johnson Foundation, the William T. Grant Foundation, and the Turrell Fund, to name just a few whose generosity in supporting our basic research program has enabled me to write this book. David Carver, as I have come to expect, continues his support of my efforts, seeing with a wide perspective the needs of children and families.

As always, my life with Rhoda Lewis has given me the vision of a just world and the need to see the connection between theory and practice.

Contents

Chapter 1

CHANCE AND NECESSITY

Everything existing in the Universe is the fruit of chance
and of necessity.
                                                    —*Democritus*

When my son, Benjamin, was very young, we used to play on the beach. The game we played was called Generations. We built a wall at the ocean's edge, and inside the wall we built a castle. The waves beat against the walls, and eventually they tore at the castle, destroying parts of it. The game involved a succession of people—parents, then children—who built and rebuilt the walls and the castle as they were destroyed by the waves. My thought behind this game was to show Benjamin the idea of generations—that each individual in his place was part of a succession, a point along a line that had no clear beginning and no end. We both enjoyed the game, but even more we enjoyed the fact that for five generations there had been a Ben and a Michael succeeding each other.

   I was teaching Benjamin the idea of development: that change was slow but inexorable, that there was direction—from parent to child to parent again. These ideas, too, he learned in our game. Much as my father had formed the child, so would I. That we played such a game was no surprise since I was myself deeply involved in trying to understand, in a more formal way, the process of development. From the beginning of my studies I took as my starting point the idea that development was a sequence of small progressions, that it had directionality and an end point, and that it was causal; that is, earlier events were connected to later ones.

This was no ideal thought of mine. From the beginning of its study, the developmental process has been understood as a unidirectional bounded process of change leading to some goal called *maturity*, where earlier events are related to later events and therefore later events can be predicted from them. This idea about development has often been called the *organismic model.*[*] The theories of both Sigmund Freud and, later, Jean Piaget follow such a model. Over the years the difficulties with this model of development have been raised, the most serious of which have to do with the concept of progress, the model's failure to consider accidents and chance, and the fact that humans have consciousness and therefore can plan their futures as well as reconstruct their pasts, all in the service of adaptation to their environments. Nevertheless, and in spite of this complexity, many people have believed, and many still do, that the developmental process is lawful and regular, that it can be studied and, with patience, understood. We certainly act as if it is so.

While earlier in my study of development I believed that a predictable, lawful process of change could be articulated, I have more recently, although with some difficulty, come to the conclusion that the study of change is in fact the study of complex emergent connections, often random, certainly unpredictable. Because of these inescapable facts, I offer in place of the organismic model of development what William James called the *pragmatic model*[2] and what I refer to here as *contextualism*, to use Stephen Pepper's term. A contextual model does not require progress or that early events necessarily are connected to later ones; it requires only adaptation to current context. This other model may not be any more demonstrable than the organismic model, and it is not my intention to refute one in favor of the other. Rather, this book's goal is to show that the problems inherent in the organismic model make contextualism worthy of greater consideration, especially since our social policy in regard to children's needs and how to parent are determined largely by the organismic view. Considering the often dismal success rates of our social intervention, the need to review the merits of another model of development is obvious.

Our social policy is founded on the belief that intervention in the lives of children who are at risk for developmental failures can alter their fate and that earlier intervention is more effective than later interven-

---

[*]I use this term in a more literary than a philosophical sense. For a more precise definition, see Overton and Reese and Reese and Overton. My use of *organismic* captures some features they have reserved for mechanistic models.[1]

tion. Years ago I visited a program in Philadelphia designed to foster the socioemotional development of children of teenage inner-city mothers. The program consisted of placing the naked newborn child on the naked belly of the child's mother in the hope that successful early bonding between the two would inoculate the child against the demands of the environment. This early action would alter the child's potentially dysfunctional developmental course.

Consider what this type of intervention means. Even though this child will live in a poverty environment often filled with violence, drugs, and disease and will be raised by a mother with little schooling and no job, the act of bonding will both affect infant and mother *now* and affect what happens *later* in life. But if we acknowledge the existence of radical discontinuities—of obstacles, chance encounters, and unavoidable accidents—it is hard to believe this intervention could be effective. It has not been. Yet social policy embedded in the idea of continuity leads to these types of intervention.

I believe that continuing to formulate social policy according to a questionable developmental model may harm our efforts to help children live the kinds of lives we wish for them. The contextual or pragmatic model, following William James's idea that the task of people is to adapt to their current environment, argues that current context is more instrumental than past events in controlling how people act in the present. There is no predictive necessity in this model. It is more like the study of history. We are better able to explain how our pasts arrived in the present than predict our futures. Translated into social policy, this means we should think of care, not cure.

Simon Schama, the historian, believes that it is the narrative of any story, the social construction, that becomes a historical truth rather than what actually occurs. In his 1991 book *Dead Certainties*, he writes that, to understand historical events,

> whether in the construction of a legend, or the execution of a crime, surely requires the telling of stories, . . . and if in the end we must be satisfied with nothing more than broken lines of communication to the past . . . we stumble only on "unimaginable accidents," and our flickering glimpses of dead worlds fall far short of ghostly immersion, that perhaps is still enough to be going on with.[3]

The same may be said of the development of a human life.

This book, therefore, is not about how humans develop; rather it is about how we think humans develop. Indeed, we do not know how humans develop even though as adults we have gone through at least some of the process and have watched our children and grandchildren go through some of it as well. Development takes place before we know what has happened; one day each of us awakes as a teenager, then as a husband, wife, lover, then as a parent, and before long we have grown old. For the last hundred years scientists have tried to study this process formally, but, in no small sense, all that has really been done is to give words and descriptions to the seasons of our lives: neonates, infants, toddlers, children, adolescents, young adults, adults, middle age, and old age.

I believe most of us still hold to these ideas about development: change is gradual and continuous; it has direction and an end point so that we can talk about progress toward that point; earlier events cause or are the precursors of later events, and in this chain of events those that occur earlier have the most impact. Don't we all believe that what happened in our childhood affects us still?

These ideas that we hold so dearly are in direct opposition to what we know about our lives and those of others. We all realize that life is dangerous and capricious. A potentially huge number of people and events can intervene in our lives, throwing us off course, redirecting our destiny. How, then, can the events of childhood be expected to maintain such a tenacious hold on us? Accidents, wars, famines, disease, and chance encounters have always been our bedfellows. These unexpected and unpredictable events punctuate our lives and should cause us to question why we think that life is a connected, predictable, steady, and orderly succession of events. Nevertheless, most of us are able to maintain both views and if questioned would still believe in the predictable model of development over any other possibility. Why do we hold to this organismic view, and why do we believe there is ample evidence to support it?

I hope to show that our choice of predictability and order is part of a larger need we have for explaining ourselves. Our need for identity, that "I remain me no matter what," takes precedence over all other possibilities. This is what fuels our strong belief in the predictable, gradual, and orderly progression of life. This is seen in our faith in epidemiology, which seeks to explain the incidence of disease and therefore tries to predict its causes from earlier events. Likewise our belief in evolution, which we understand as a sequence of gradual and steady changes. Or in our fascination with biographies and autobiographies, which try to explain how famous people get to be the way they are.

In a recent article in *Science* entitled "Epidemiology Faces Its Limits,"[4] Gary Taubes writes about the difficulties in searching for the relation between what we eat, drink, breathe, and where we live—such as near toxic dumps—and disease. The epidemiological argument rests on the fact that genetic factors cannot explain the change in the rate of a disease or differences among populations; for example, the rates of heart disease change too fast to be explained by genetic changes, and no single cancer affects all populations equally. Epidemiology holds that earlier events, such as where we lived or what we ate, affect later events. But can we show that earlier events cause later ones? Taubes notes the great difficulty epidemiologists have in finding answers to the questions they pose. In fact, the title of the review article gives it away—"its limits." Besides a few accepted associations between earlier and later events such as cigarette smoking and lung cancer, or sunlight and skin cancer, little else is really known. Even so, we are continually informed about the latest association, only to discover a year or so later that what we thought was true often is not. For example, reserpine, which was used for the control of high blood pressure, was thought to cause a fourfold increase in the risk of breast cancer. The findings were wrong, but the drug disappeared anyway. The risk of a high serum cholesterol level has been well publicized, but new findings suggest that the level of cholesterol is less important than the ratio of high-density lipoproteins (HDL) to total cholesterol.

These problems will continue to arise because epidemiological studies look for an association between earlier and later events. These studies are invariably thwarted by the complexity of the unfolding of change. Any event is embedded in a large set of other events, and it is not easy to separate out the particular event in question. People who smoke also are apt to drink more alcohol and are likely to be poorer than those who do not smoke. The neighborhoods they live in are different from those inhabited by nonsmokers, and they are exposed to different environmental risks, like carbon dioxide and lead. This covarying set of events means that there are many possible causes of a later event like cancer. While it might be possible to show statistically the effect of a particular event, it is *not* possible to identify all of the covarying factors, and thus it is not possible to claim cause.

Even when epidemiologists find an association, say between smoking and lung cancer, it is clear that not every person who smokes gets cancer. That is, while epidemiologists can tell us that smokers are four times more likely to develop lung cancer than nonsmokers, they cannot tell us who in particular will get it. The interaction and covariation of a complex set of events are likely to mean that we can do no better than an estimate for the general population. For cigarettes that may be good enough.

Along with the problem of covarying events comes the problem of change. While diet, for example, may be related to subsequent illness, we know little about the timing involved. For example, what if I ate red meat for twenty years and then stopped? Would stopping have the same effect as not having eaten red meat at all? Given the combination of factors and the timing issue, the study of epidemiology may be restricted to only a few highly associated events.

Nevertheless, we continue to believe that we can predict. We greet each new finding as if it is real, and we alter our behavior according to it. In the last decade in this country we have significantly reduced our consumption of red meat, eggs, alcohol, and cigarettes, reduced our weight, and increased our exercise, all under the belief that we will avoid disease and live longer. Our behavior manifests a commitment to the belief that earlier events cause later ones and that we can predict the association between them.

To study the etiology of disease for an individual is, admittedly, to look at change within a small time frame. Nevertheless, our ideas about development do not differ when placed inside a larger time frame. Anyone who knows anything about Charles Darwin's theory of evolution knows that change is gradual and continual and that natural selection—the survival of the fittest—rules. Despite widespread acceptance, however, the idea of gradual and continuous change is now being challenged. Recently, Alan Cheetham presented data on bryozoans, corallike animals with a fifteen-million-year-old fossil record, the most intact record found to date. Based on the data, Cheetham stated, "I came reluctantly to the conclusion that I wasn't finding evidence for gradualism."[5] Cheetham and his collaborator, Jeremy Jackson, have rejected gradualism in evolutionary biology and confirmed the idea of punctuated equilibrium.

The theory of punctuated equilibrium was first proposed nearly twenty-five years ago by Niles Eldredge and Stephen Jay Gould, who held to the idea that evolutionary history consists of periods of status or no change as well as periods of sudden change. Since Darwin, paleontologists have attributed the lack of evidence for gradualism to flaws in the geological record, but this new theory of sudden change appears to account more adequately for the development of species. Also supporting the idea of sudden change, either in species creation or in extinction, is the theory that a meteor struck the earth, producing a thick cloud layer enshrouding the globe and leading ultimately to the destruction of the dinosaurs.

Sudden change occurs, and the reasons for it are unclear. What is clear, at least from the extinction of some species, is that sudden change can be caused by events outside the system. These events are likely to be random to the developmental process itself. They are accidents and chance encounters. They make efforts at prediction seem impossible. Yet, in spite of what we know, we still believe in gradualism and predicting the future.

Biography also is an attempt at understanding how earlier events predict later lives. Biographers take the information about a life and try to construct its causal history. They write that this event, often something in early childhood, is related to—causes and therefore can be used as a predictor of—later ones. It is like a puzzle, where life events lying on the table are put together in some reasonable order, always with an eye to explaining why lives are as they are.

In a recent article in *The New Yorker* Ron Rosenbaum[6] reviewed the efforts of those trying to put together the puzzle of Adolf Hitler's life. In "Explaining Hitler," Rosenbaum looks at the two chief authors who have devoted themselves to trying to understand the early conditions that formed this person.

Both Hugh Trevor-Roper and Alan Bullock conclude that the causes of Hitler's monstrous actions remain a confusing mystery. This is because the reasons the biographer gives for an outcome are varied and are determined largely by general beliefs that the historian holds. In the case of Hitler, the beliefs range from unconscious urges to mental confusion, the absence of his left testicle, a dose of syphilis, his discovery that he had been fathered by a Jew, the death of his mother at the hands of a Jewish doctor, his interest in pornography, his reading of tales of lustful Jews using sexual exploration to defile German maidens, his having been hypnotized to cure his blindness from poisonous gas, violent beatings at the hands of his father, and finally incestuousness toward his mother. As we can see, the earlier causes of Hitler's actions seem unlimited. As Rosenbaum writes: "One paradox in attempting to explain Hitler is that there are already too many explanations. A tour of the literature of Hitler theories . . . can yield the impression that Hitler's crimes were the most overdetermined events in history. . . ."[7] The reconstruction of such a life is difficult not only because there are too many facts to explain but also because some facts always remain unknown. But given that we could know all the facts, how could we know how they go together? Do our theories come from the facts, or do we use the facts to justify our theories? I believe that the facts, even if they were all known, would not order themselves into a causal chain. What they require is a story line, a narrative or way to fit them together. It is our need for the narrative that orders the events and lends belief to their causal nature.

A recently published biography of Edward O. Wilson underscores how elusive predictability is and how important it is for each of us to explain our life. Wilson wrote his story "to understand how . . . [the] apparently unlikely connections [between events] make sense in hindsight."[8] A world-renowned biologist, Wilson's early life reads like the story of a man who would not amount to anything. His family background was uneducated—none had ever gone to college. He came from a divorced family with an alcoholic father who committed suicide. He suffered many physical ailments, including mild hearing loss and near blindness in one eye. Moreover, he was a poor student. When asked, few of us would predict that such a history would lead to a distinguished academic career. In fact, we often use circumstances such as lack of education in the family background, early parental death, divorce, and alcoholism as examples of the possible causes of poor school or work performance. Yet Wilson did succeed, and his autobiography is an attempt to explain how this came about. Is it a true explanation or just a good story? How can we know?

Many of us would argue that for both of these lives there was some predetermined path that accounted for their particular outcomes. Something in these men, a trait found early, determined that they were to be evil or successful. No matter what particular challenge or random event occurred, this trait would always lead them back to their predetermined path. Thus, while Wilson confronted many challenges, the traits he possessed allowed him always to come out right.

Such an argument would have us believe that accidents and chance encounters influence us only as long as we let them. Letting them implies a process that itself is influenced by our pasts and that allows only certain events and not others to affect us. The belief that early events affect later behavior is as ingrown, as fixed, as certain as any idea we have concerning human life.

The history of such a belief can be found in many areas of thought, and it seems as if we have always believed it true. Freud's earliest writing in *The Interpretation of Dreams*[9] deals with determinism and accidents. For Freud, accidents, slips of the tongue, and dreams are deterministic and have meaning. He argued against randomness. Nothing in our psychic lives is random, he believed. If there are no accidents, if dreams or slips of the tongue or even hurting oneself has a cause located in our early experiences, then the idea that chance or accidents can determine lives is much deflated. I can think of nothing more powerful than the idea that there is no such thing as an accident or a slip of the tongue to support the argument for determinism based on early experience.

In more modern times, the idea of personality has come to dominate our view of human behavior. Personality can be considered the relatively fixed nature of behavior in the face of changing situations. We see ourselves as having a set of fixed traits that are likely to lead us to behave, think, or feel the same way no matter what the situation we find ourselves in.[10] The idea of a fixed personality is very potent and powerful. At its heart is the claim that traits exist and so future behavior can be determined if we understand what they are.

A decade ago, Albert Bandura wrote a paper entitled "The Psychology of Chance Encounters and Life Paths" in which he said, "Psychological theories have neglected the fundamental issue of what determines people's life paths. The central thesis . . . is that chance encounters play a prominent role in shaping the course of human lives."[11] Such an idea, when introduced into the study of development, must force us to reflect on the possibility that development is a series of changes best understood by looking backward and accounting for what has transpired rather than looking forward to predict what will occur.

Edward Wilson's attempt to make plausible the connections between his early life and how it has come out forms his narrative. These life narratives, a way for us to account for and put in order the events of our lives, are important to all of us since they provide us with a story of and an explanation for why we are the way we are. These narratives carry our identity; they explain to us and to others what we are by accounting for how that came about. Their importance for people is not whether they are correct but whether the story they tell is satisfying.

In the chapters to follow, I will question the claim of such narratives that these earlier events in our lives have somehow caused our later behavior. While the narratives are important in their own right, I also question their veracity since they rest on our memories of our past. As we shall see, memories of the past themselves serve our current narrative. We remember or even reconstruct memories that fit with what we think about ourselves now.[12] Our reconstructions of our past and how they lead to what we are now are at best only explanations. The causal path forward in time—the prediction of the future given the past—is complex.

As I have suggested, the complexity of causes, the number of events, and interaction over time make it difficult to predict the course of human life. But there is even more. The problem that applies to evolutionary time also applies to a human life: random events outside our lives—wars, famine, disease, accidents, and deaths—act on our lives. Like the meteor that crashed into earth, they are all capable of altering our lives in unimaginable ways, and they occur around us all the time. Even the genes we are born with mutate and in their change alter our lives. In my own life, even as I tried to study the orderliness of change, I encountered them. In fact, reflecting on personal experience almost inevitably leads to the conclusion that life is not gradual and predictable but that random accidents may be more the rule than the exception.

Complexity, multiple determination, accidents, and chance encounters are just some of the problems inherent in the study of development. What I have left for last in the study of people's lives is the problem of consciousness, the fact that we are not merely grains of sand or laboratory rats but creatures who can think and are capable of thinking about ourselves. Having consciousness means that we can think about the past, present, and future, that we can plan, desire, and have a moral sense. Consciousness allows us to separate the past from the present and the present from the future. We can alter our lives by wishing, hoping, planning, and remembering. Consciousness allows us to try to predict our lives as well as to intervene in altering the events that have not yet happened.

It is, as I will discuss later in the book, what makes us human, what separates us from other animals. It is also why I chose to title this book *Altering Fate*. If we are to understand how we think humans develop, we must accept the idea that models allowing for prediction also seal our fate. What we need is a model that has as its principle current adaptation and, as such, allows for altering fate, something we do every day.

To intervene when we observe suffering and injustice is obviously good. To do so expecting to have a particular effect on the future may be folly because we—and other forces over which we have no control—alter our fate in unpredictable ways every day. If the examples given so far represent the reality of lives, then our notions about development are too simple. We need to change them. To change them requires that we understand as best we can why we hold a gradual, orderly, progressive, connected, and causal view of development. The model that depicts development as a trajectory, undisturbed by surrounding events, although created from those events earlier in time, needs reconsideration. I propose that in its place we consider the idea of contextualism, an idea that does not require historicism.* Individuals develop in the presence of random events, and lives are more characterized by zigs and zags than by some predetermined, connected, and linear pattern. It is only when we understand how organisms are influenced by their environments *now* and how their ideas that exist *now* for their futures can affect their desires and behaviors that we can understand the nature of development, how we got to be what we are, and how we might go about making a more perfect and just society, both for ourselves and for those who are less fortunate than we.

Aristotle thought there were two kinds of facts: *to oti*, or a fact in itself, and *di oti*, or a reasoned fact. I should like to argue that development as a gradual, continuous, causally related sequence, where early events affect later ones, is in fact only a *to oti*. It is simply a fact in itself; a belief that we have. Moreover, it is a relatively new belief. What we need to do is to produce a *di oti*, a reasoned fact. If we are successful, we can be so only to the degree that the reader is prepared, at least for a moment, to suspend the idea of development as a *di oti*.[13]

OVERVIEW

The ideas I have introduced in this chapter may seem far from revolutionary: Accidents happen; chance is real. When we least expect it, something or someone comes along to alter our lives. How, then, is it possible for both scientist and layperson to cling to a model of develop-

---

*Although Hayne W. Reese believes continuity is contextual and discontinuity organismic, these associations appear strained and contradict standard meaning. It need not be so if contexts themselves are not continuous!

ment that does not acknowledge these aspects of the human condition? The answer, I believe, lies in the fixity of certain ideas that underlie our basic beliefs. These ideas not only affect what we believe but determine how we parent and how the society's social policies, in regard to children's health and welfare, are carried out. In Chapter 2 I discuss several fixed ideas that combine to form a world view common to Western culture, a view that both supports and derives from the organismic model of development. I begin my challenge of the organismic model by challenging these underlying fixed ideas: the idea of continuity, that people are the passive slaves to their own pasts, that the past is real and acts on the present.

Whether one accepts continuity and the other fixed ideas discussed in Chapter 2 will determine which of the two competing models of development, presented in Chapters 3 and 4, one accepts. In Chapter 3, "Traditional Models of Change," I explain exactly how the organismic model works and describe possible alternatives so that the assumptions underlying the model can be examined. Chapter 4, "Development in Context," presents the contextual model of development, a model that does not require continuity, gradualism, or historicism. Here William James's idea of pragmaticism and Stephen Pepper's contextualism combine with Darwin's ideas of development as random change and adaptation to the current situation. Here, too, we see that the organismic model of development allows us to predict the next five minutes but has little use in predicting development over time. In addition, development appears to have no clear directionality—the past is explained by the present as well as the past predicting the present—which means that a linear, causal, and directional process called organismic development may not readily be found.

If development is not unidirectional, the utopian concept of progress that underlies the organismic model of change is called into question. In Chapter 5, "Progress and the Metaphor of Development," I explore the metaphor of the organismic model that progress is a part of development and that there exists some idealized end point to life. This still-active metaphor harbors two inescapable problems: first, the child never *is* but is always *becoming*; second, since there is progress, what comes later is a better or higher form of being, meaning that the child is an inadequate adult rather than a very adequate child. These ideas affect how we behave toward children. The idea of progress is a dream invented to lead us always forward. It needs to be reviewed.

In all discussions about the developmental process, the issue of the meaning of behavior is central. The ability to follow the course of lives is feasible only if we can understand the meaning of the behaviors we study. In Chapter 6, "Behavior Serves Many Masters," I present one of my earliest and perhaps longest and strongest held beliefs: given that meaning is assigned not by the observer but by the subjects themselves, the ability to understand the meaning of behavior remains doubtful. Behavior has meaning only as it is embedded in the present context, and the continuity of behavior over time has little use. Measurement error cannot be used as an excuse for why we cannot predict development over time.

The measurement problem informs us that no observation of a process, without taking into account the self's perspective of that process, can provide anything but the experimenter's idea as to what is happening. The idea that meaning resides not in the observer or the interaction between observer and observed but in that which is observed rests on Isaac Newton's classical idea of the universe. Newton believed that the universe was like a gigantic clock that could be opened and observed without disturbing it. Psychology, utilizing the image of modern science, accepted this metaphor in spite of the fact that twentieth-century quantum mechanics and the theory of relativity have altered this view of the nature of reality. Relativity has replaced the absolute. Chapter 7, "Newton, Einstein, Piaget, and the Self," addresses this epistemological issue. Here I address the limitations of Jean Piaget's developmental theory and consider the need to take the knower into account in explaining the development of intelligence. More specifically, I illustrate Piaget's lack in not bringing the subject into clearer focus by comparing his view with Albert Einstein's relativistic approach. Empathy provides a good case study of the different views. The ability to place the self in the role of the other is contrasted to egocentric thought to show that the known cannot be separated from the self as knower. The changing view of the nature of inquiry gives rise to my particular interest in the individual who works behind the process and whose action I study but do not understand. This quality of consciousness helps to explain why the study of development is so difficult and, at the same time, how we might attempt to study it in the future. The self as knower and the reiterative quality of such knowledge, for me, explain in part why a predictive science of development may not be possible.

The failure to consider the self in knowing is related to the issue of consciousness, a topic considered in Chapter 8, "Consciousness and

Being." While we might think that any theory of development would have to take consciousness into account, the organismic view allows us to think of people as controlled by their pasts. The theory has little use for an active person, one capable of learning from mistakes and thus altering the future by changing the past. It is consciousness that allows us to separate past from future. A conscious self fits well into the contextual model, which holds that one of our major tasks is to explain ourselves, to create a historical narrative that allows for the maintenance of our identity, and to plan for the future. The consciousness aspect of ourselves, as this chapter discusses, emerges in the early years and allows children to participate in their own development. Almost from the beginning people know about themselves, and this knowledge allows them to alter their lives.

The contextual model of development gives rise to the need to understand the nature of the environment in which the child grows. The environment deserves the same attention as does the child's behavior. We cannot understand behavior without studying behavior-in-context. Perhaps the most serious consequence of following the organismic model of development is in the study of children's socioemotional development. Attachment theory is a prime example of the organismic theory applied to emotional and social development. In Chapter 9, "Adaptation and the Nature of Social Life," I explore the two most prominent theories about the child's social environment: the family system versus the attachment model. The attachment model, proposed by John Bowlby, is in most respects the same organismic model as that expounded by Freud, and an important part of it is the belief that only one person, the child's mother, early in the child's life, is important to the child's development. I wish to argue that the social network, including but not restricted to the mother, at any point in time creates a set of challenges that requires us to adapt. Adaptation is a continuous process since environments change, change that occurs both by chance and by our earlier adaptive responses.

Chapter 10, "Time, Sudden Change, and Catastrophe," brings us back to the concept of chance introduced earlier in this chapter, focusing on the difficulties inherent in any study of change as a continuous and gradual process. If catastrophe is a property of change regardless of the nature of that change, then human development should occur within that constraint, and the unexpected, the chaotic, the unpredictable, and the accidental all are likely. The idea of catastrophe is considered, because it has a role in the history of the planet and in the unfolding of life as we know it. If not for catastrophe, we would expect the course of the destruction of species to be uniform. Instead we see catastrophic moments in time, geological epochs, as they are called, when large numbers of species appear and disappear. Thus, geological and evolutionary time is marked by catastrophe. At the human level, we need to accept the idea that catastrophe, rather than steady, gradual, and orderly change, characterizes the lives of people and that these random moments inexorably alter the smooth and predictable course of development. Chance encounters, unavoidable accidents, and the whims of others, all random events external to the individual, as well as the chaotic moments of transformation within individuals themselves, lead us to understand that what has happened will inform us at best only in a limited way of what is likely to happen in the future.

In the last chapter, "Cure or Care," the contrasts between the organismic and contextual models are shown to interact with our hopes for social change and the role of values in creating a just society. Because so much of our policy is based on the idea of an organismic pattern of development—a continuous, predictable process moving to an end point where earlier events are likely to produce later events—rather than on a contextualist theory in which current behavior and needs may not be related to past events but to present adaptation, it is important that we review how social policy might differ if our model of development were changed. To anticipate the argument, I will suggest that social policy needs to be designed to prevent subsequent dysfunction in children and families but, more important, to provide for their current needs. In some sense, then, our policy of intervention at one point in time, with the expectation that it should positively affect development at a subsequent point in time, needs to give way to a model in which intervention is applied at all points in time. The idea of cure must give way to the idea of care!

Simply put, in these eleven chapters I wish to argue against the idea that development is a sequence of small progressions that are gradual but accumulative, that it has clear directionality, that it is causal—earlier events are connected to later ones—and that prediction therefore is possible. Instead, I would like to argue for the idea that development is based on the pragmatic needs of the present, that the contextual flow of our lives determines our development through adaptation to the current. As a people and a nation, we may have too much invested in a single model of development. If I am at all successful, it will be in providing a new framework in which to view our social intervention strategies as we seek to build a more just, happier, and healthier society.

Chapter 2

T HREE FIXED IDEAS

————————

T ime and space are absolute. Diseases are evil spirits that inhabit the body. Parallel lines never meet. The earth is the center of the universe. Children are miniature adults.

At one time in history each of these beliefs was generally held to be true. Each, however, gave way to different ideas and even different world views. If we were to discover that beneath our widely accepted theories of human development there were fixed ideas and world views that should be questioned, we would not hesitate to do so. If these fixed ideas led to social policies designed to cure the ills of society that were not working, our task would be to speak loudly to these fallacies.

In French *idée fixe* means an idea that is fixed in the mind, one that holds a special place and cannot easily be dislodged. No amount of evidence to the contrary can alter it. In psychiatry a fixed idea is a pathology of sorts; in common parlance it has come to mean obsession. In philosophy a group of fixed ideas is called a *world view,* similar to the term *world hypothesis* coined by Stephen C. Pepper fifty years ago.[1] A world view is a set of ideas about how things work or why things are the way they are. In a sense world views are like the axioms in Euclidean geometry, a set of ideas on which all other ideas are built. Although the wide and complex set of interconnected ideas and beliefs based on these axioms can be tested, the axioms themselves cannot be proven or disproven. For example, the world view of many people includes the belief in a personal God, one who hears our supplications and intervenes in our lives. No one has ever been able to prove that such a God exists or does not exist. That does not mean, however, that prevailing beliefs about God have never changed. In the Western world alone, the Greek pantheon ultimately gave way to the monotheistic Judeo-Christian tradition (with various detours along the way). Euclidean geometry eventually gave up some ground to the non-Euclidean geometries of N. I. Lobachevski, G. F. B. Riemann, and company.

The information we scientists gather should be understood as it applies to a world view. Our world views affect how we measure things, what we measure, and how we interpret what we find. To understand human development and the information collected to study change, we need to understand the world views that underlie our theories.

Many of our beliefs about development are related to what has been called by some the *organismic model*. In turn the organismic model rests on particular ideas. How we stand in regard to these ideas determines for the most part if we accept this model or choose its alternative, which I will call the *contextualist model*. These ideas are (1) continuity or discontinuity; (2) the issue of will, or the active versus the passive view of human behavior; and (3) history as photograph or as narrative. While it may be impossible to prove without a doubt which stance on these three issues is correct, it is certainly possible to see how the opposing beliefs hold up to a test of logic and what kind of data are available to support them. Should we discover cracks in these foundations, we must conclude that the models of development on which they stand are shaky indeed.

CONTINUITY OR DISCONTINUITY

I am sitting in a garden where I can see flowers around me. Each day the flowers grow. Let's say I focus my attention on a single flower—a daffodil—and every day I watch its growth. I see the leaves appear first, followed by the stem, then the flower. For several days the bloom remains vibrant. One morning I look again and the bloom has wilted. I have witnessed birth, growth, and death, the process of change. Because the flower grows too slow for my moment-to-moment perception, how might I say I watched it grow? If I looked once each hour and took a picture of what I saw, at the end of the week I would have one hundred sixty-eight pictures. Each of the pictures would be discrete, and yet my response as I watched the flower grow and as I look across the set of pictures I have collected is to a gradual and continuous process of change. What if I took sixty pictures a minute rather than one an hour? Then, at the end of a week, I would have 604,800 pictures. Each one of these pictures represents a discrete moment; yet, again, if I could move quickly through them, I would experience the flower growing in a continuous fashion.

We all know that continuity appears to exist even in the presence of discontinuity. Vary the speed on a movie projector or a reel-to-reel tape recorder. Individual frames become a moving picture only when they are moving too fast for the eye to perceive the breaks between them; discrete notes become a hum and then a squeal the faster the music is played. Throughout history people have been fascinated with the fact that continuity and discontinuity apparently coexist and have struggled to understand which one really explains the way things work. Everett Mendelson, for example, in his analysis of the history of science, suggests that the debate over continuous versus discontinuous change goes back as far as Aristotle and his distaste for the atomism of Leucippus and Democritus.[2]

In the ensuing millennia the idea that change is continuous has generally held sway. In theories of development it is at the core of the organismic model, and it is not difficult to understand why people tend to favor it over discontinuity. The idea of continuity fills our lives and gives them meaning. It is the way we experience ourselves and our world, a framework for the way we look at our past, present, and future. Without continuity it would be meaningless to talk about what we did yesterday, how it makes us feel today, and how it may change our plans for tomorrow. No wonder then that an organismic model of development has been so easy to accept. It is the conviction that life is "an uninterrupted connection or succession" or a "stretching on without break or interruption" that has led so many developmental psychologists to try to predict how earlier events in a child's life influence later ones. Without the element of continuity, no one would propose what psychotherapists informed by the organismic model state as if it were fact: that how our mothers treated us will affect our married lives.

In the study of human lives we look at continuity in terms of two ideas that grow out of the definitions I just quoted: *uninterruption*, or nonseparation between parts, and the *connection* of those parts, most often referring to the belief that earlier events are connected to later ones. A third, closely related idea is the concept of *gradualism*. Not included in dictionary definitions of continuity, the idea of gradualism, or progression, is nonetheless inextricably connected to the concepts of uninterruption and connection—at least in developmental theory. In the abstract, continuity need not imply gradualism; an uninterrupted connection or succession could be made up of large units without break. Because we are observing how a human being—or any other organism for that matter—develops over time, however, continuity and gradualism are seen together more often than not.

In fact, however, the more we study continuity in nature, the more the existence of discontinuities is impressed on us. The idea of "discontinuity may disappear and be smoothed down at one point," wrote John Theodore Merz early in this century in an examination of nineteenth-century thought, "only to reappear again in a more mysterious manner at other points."[3] We know, for instance, that the apparently continuous physical growth of children is in fact made up of a set of very small jumps. Children grow a bit daily, not all day long but only at night.

Based on data alone, there is little support for the argument that continuity best characterizes development. So far it has been difficult to show that earlier events in people's lives are related to or connected to later ones, and a perusal of works published in recent years shows that others who have addressed this subject have found little evidence to support the argument for continuity.[4]

Part of the problem rests on the difficulty in measuring continuity, a subject taken up later in this book. What is pertinent now is that although no data can prove or disprove that discontinuity is the rule, in every aspect of life and every field of science I see it "reappear in a more mysterious manner," as Merz said. The continuity–discontinuity issue touches on evolutionary theory, physics, and even political ideology; its pervasiveness is brought up in almost every chapter of this book.

If continuity is so questionable, then so are the social policy and social intervention strategies founded on it. We need to explore therefore how the theme of continuity impacts on our common beliefs about how events in our lives are connected and how we apply those beliefs in setting policy for social action. The purpose of my arguments in subsequent chapters is to show that discontinuity is as real as continuity. If discontinuity is to be our model, it will lead to a very different set of social policies aimed at children, families, and societies.

THE ISSUE OF WILL

A second issue underlying our understanding of the nature of development is that of will, the role of people in their own development. Are we active or passive organisms? Most of our ideas about development and the studies that inform our view treat children as passive agents influenced by forces that determine their developmental course. Our Western creation myth is our central model of passivity.* Like Adam, formed from clay, children are formed from the biological material of which they are made or by the hands of their parents.

The first of these forces can be described as the biological imperative: the child's developmental course is the consequence of biological processes inherent in the genome. We know, for example, that as children get older they generally get taller and heavier. While it is true that they have to eat for this growth to take place, the eating simply supplies the material to allow a biological process to take place. The child is passive.

The biological imperative to varying degrees is said to determine development, both the structures and the processes that underlie the sequence of change. Under this passive model all the child can do is try to interfere with the process. The child may choose not to eat, for example, which will interfere with gains in height and weight. But the fact that the child can take this active role, even if it is a negative one, in the face of a strong biological imperative suggests that human beings cannot be viewed as purely passive organisms in their own development.

The second powerful imperative controlling children's development is the social environment. Children are treated as if they are simply putty, each individual an amorphous and undefined mass that needs to be shaped by the environment, the child's behavior determined by outside forces. Perhaps the most obvious example of this is the operant reinforcement theory of B. F. Skinner.[5] In Skinner's view, a child's behavior is shaped by the rewards and punishments of the social environment. Parents get their children to do things by rewarding them for doing them or by punishing the children for not doing them. An extreme version of this environmental imperative can be seen in the child-rearing practices Lawrence Stone describes in *The Family, Sex, and Marriage in England, 1500 to 1800*.[6] These practices deliberately sought to break down the

---

*It should be noted that in the Hebrew original there are two stories, one where Adam and Eve are passive recipients of God's creation and one where they participate in the creation—that is, they are created first by God and with Him name the animals as they are created. Needless to say, this part of the myth was not incorporated into the most commonly held creation myth as found in the King James version of the Bible.

child's will in the name of socializing the child. It was deemed the key to good parenting.

This practice is still in vogue according to *For Your Own Good*, a book in which Alice Miller reviews these parenting techniques and attacks this idea. "Therefore, I advise all those whose concern is the education of children," Miller quotes from a child-rearing manual,

> to make it their main occupation to drive out willfulness and wickedness, and to persist until they have reached their goal. . . . It is impossible to reason with young children; thus, willfulness must be driven out in a methodological manner, and there is no other recourse for this purpose than to show children what is serious.[7]

The manual Miller quotes from is one hundred fifty years old, yet a surprising number of modern parents would still consider it appropriate for raising children today!

How strong the belief is that children should not participate in their own development can be seen in attitudes toward conceit, Miller explains. Conceit, it seems, causes children to think they are capable of making decisions. Miller goes on to report an example of this attitude:

> Conceit frequently hinders a pedagogue's effectiveness; the conceited pupil believes he already possesses the good qualities the pedagogue teaches and expects of him, or at least considers them easily attainable. Warnings he deems signs of exaggerated apprehensiveness—words of censure, signs of peevish severity. Only humiliation can be of help here.[8]

These ideas make it clear that for the Western mind the prevailing view of successful child rearing has changed less over the last four hundred years than we may think: due to the evil nature of children, adults must train them harshly, first to make the child passive and then to inculcate the correct material.

Today's enlightened parents will undoubtedly protest, citing nonpunitive approaches now used widely in education and child management. Yet close examination of these practices reveals that they still assume children are passive in the process. A child's right to have a will and to assert it may now be acknowledged, but how often do adults allow the child to *act* on that will? Also, parents who believe that they harbor no vestige of the attitude that children are inherently evil might find it revealing to recall what they often think about an adolescent son or daughter. Psychoanalytic theory keeps this malicious-child model from fading away altogether by clinging to the Freudian view that children are full of evil impulses residing in the id and that it is the task of the parents to control these impulses. Freud viewed children as reluctant and often negative factors in their own development. Parents and the socializing society had the task of converting, suppressing, and transforming these evil impulses into structures useful to society, first ego functions and later the superego or moral functions. More recent theorists stress parental love and empathy as sources for the child's proper development, but here again the view remains that the child is acted on and altered by these actions.

There is, of course, an alternative view—that children are active participants in their own socialization and development.[9] Rather than being subjected to forces that impact on them, children can be viewed as eager, willing, and capable organisms who possess the ability to create and change their behavior to meet the demands of a social system and the biological imperatives that arise. Social control and biological imperatives can be seen not as controlling forces but rather as input that informs children about their own nature and the nature of their environment. With this knowledge, children then are capable of constructing how to behave and what to think. Consider the case where a child is punished or rewarded for certain types of social behavior. The child may be punished for hitting another child and grabbing the toy he wants but rewarded when he politely asks for the toy. Viewed from an active-organism perspective, the child actively uses his knowledge of which behaviors are being punished and which are being rewarded to construct a model about socially appropriate behavior and is able to generalize the rules to other situations when no reinforcement is given. He is able to create categories of meaning from which he can decide how to act. The ability to construct knowledge and alter the basis of decision making around one's own plans and goals is the hallmark of the active organism, one who has consciousness.

As with the idea of development's being either continuous or discontinuous, there is no way to argue convincingly that human beings are either completely active or completely passive. But it is not difficult to see how passive versus active lines up with continuity versus discontinuity. A pattern of gradual and connected change is likely to reflect an organism that is relatively inactive to the forces creating that change. An active organism, possessing consciousness, capable of adjusting its behavior and altering its goals, is more likely to fit into a model in which there are sudden transformations and changes in development. The ideas of continuity and a passive organism are likely to go together in one world view, while those of discontinuity and an active organism are likely to cluster in another.

HISTORY AS PHOTOGRAPH OR NARRATIVE

In *Dead Certainties*, Simon Schama presents the reader with two accounts of a historical event.[10] In the first he discusses what he calls "the many deaths of General Wolfe." Starting with the painting *General Wolfe's Death* by Benjamin West, he leads the reader through an account of the eighteenth-century battle (1759) in which General James Wolfe lost his life and, at the same time, speaks to West's depiction of Wolfe's death on the battlefield on the Plains of Abraham (above Quebec City). What he demonstrates is that Wolf died in a less heroic fashion than depicted by West. Rather than surrounded by Indians, generals, and onlookers, Wolfe died nearly alone on a dark and bloody field. The point of Schama's story is the discrepancy between what might be called the real historical event and memories and depictions of it.

Historians in general are confronted with the task of understanding history. In pursuit of their goal they sometimes forget to ask whether what actually happened and our accounts of it bear any one-to-one relation. Unfortunately, this means ignoring a truth that appears self-evident. History belongs to those who write it. Losers of battles, the dead, and the enslaved do not write histories. Why we should lose sight of such an obvious fact is unclear. Perhaps it has something to do with our desire to believe in history, to believe that events that occurred in the past are real and have influenced the present. Such a view fits with our belief in continuity, the connection of events over time. What this leaves us with is the belief that history is an accurate representation of what actually happened, a view that occupies an extremely important place in our psyches. I call this the view of *history as photograph* because we apparently believe that if we reenacted it as written we would see exactly what occurred as if it had been recorded using a camera or a video recorder.

The alternative view of history is *history as narrative*; that is, it does not represent in any one-to-one fashion what actually occurred but is rather our construction of what occurred. I see this changing narrative much like the children's game of "telephone," in which the first child whispers to the second a particular sentence—what we could think of as the initial event. The second child then repeats that statement to the third child, and so on down the line. At the end of the line, the last child gets up and recites the sentence she heard. We all remember the delight of discovering that the statement changed, often completely, in the course of its transmission. Exactly when the change took place is unclear. At one point the message might have been communicated directly, at another point there might have been a small distortion, and at another time a large distortion might have occurred. This game reflects the narrative model of history, a model that specifies only that history is influenced by those who tell it and hear it.

Obviously historians have a vested interest in convincing us that their accounts of history are accurate. Saying, "This simply is my con-struction of history and it reflects the biases of the people who have repeated it over time; I don't know what really happened," would be a good way to put themselves out of work. In spite of translation problems or changes in language, in spite of the clear biases involved in the relating of any historical event, we readers enter into a conspiracy with historians to accept as true their stories of the past.[11]

If we have such a strong bias toward our belief in history, how much truer is this about our belief in our own histories? Those asked about their memories of their past usually suggest a photographic model. Just try to suggest to someone that his memories of childhood are not true but are constructed stories designed to explain why he is as he is now. We are firmly committed to the belief that our autobi-ographies are true.

I recently had the opportunity to suggest to someone that a very clear memory she had of her early childhood was a construction. She believed that her grandmother had died in the same year as her mother and was quite angry at my suggestion that her memory of the timing might be inaccurate. When she checked the dates on the tombstones, she saw that their deaths had occurred two years apart!

People vary in how strongly they believe in personal history as a photograph. Some believe that everything is photographed and located somewhere in their brain; others argue that everything might have been photographed, that is, collected, but only certain things are retained. In the above instance, this person was shocked by her discovery because she believed, as we all do, that at least important events remain as clear in our minds as a photo sealed in plastic. To the contrary, distortion is possible even with the most powerful historical events.

Interestingly, the same problem of memory can affect whole families. Each family passes stories about the hardships and successes of family members from generation to generation. Probably all of us have an uncle, an aunt, or a grandparent who made and lost a great fortune, survived great adversity, or, through hard work and diligence, made a success of life when no one else in the family could. These family stories have the same properties as autobiographical accounts. Family members have a strong emotional commitment to such legends, and it is very difficult to convince them that the events may not have occurred.

The view of history as photograph is essential to an organismic point of view. There are, of course, different views of the role of history in child development.[12] Since the organismic and similar models of development hold that earlier events impact on later ones, events in the past must be real to the extent to which they exert influence on the present. But exactly how an earlier event interacts with a series of later events to lead to subsequent behavior is very difficult to explain, perhaps impossible. This suggests that an alternative strategy—looking at the present narrative and relating it to behavior, forgetting about whether or not this contemporaneous model bears any resemblance to something called the historical past—could be more fruitful.

The topic of attachment is a good example of this problem. John Bowlby and Mary Main and her colleagues believe that children's relationships with their mother in the early years of life (a real event) create a model or representation that impacts on subsequent life, affecting both how the grown children parent and how they relate to others in romantic relationships.[13] The first question that must be asked is, does this representation, created from the actual events, correspond to what actually happened? Second, if not, how has the representation changed? And, finally, if the representation is not a photograph of the original event, why should we study the earlier event at all? These questions suggest ultimately that what happened earlier may or may not be of any importance to the representation of it held later. If this is the case, then from a theoretical point of view the opening year of life is relatively unimportant! Tracing how the attachment representation might change over time may be important; however, in terms of what influences the person's behavior at any given point, it is not the original event but the representation of the event that is important.

Consider what this means for social policy issues. It means it is not necessary to study children's early attachment relationships or to worry, as we do now, whether this early attachment relationship will be disrupted by such things as a mother working or the effects of day care. These considerations are important only insofar as they influence what is happening now, not what will happen in the future. Even though there might be an original one-to-one representation of what happened between the child and the mother, the subsequent transformations of that representation render the initial event relatively unimportant for the future.

To summarize my view of history, I give this quote from Klaus Riegel:

> Our inability to learn how it really was in history should disturb us as little as our failure, according to Kant, to recognize "the thing as such." History, as it really was, is hidden behind a series of interpretive filters and narratives, selectively preserved by archivists, interpreted by scholars with particular points of view, ideologies of particular times, and the difficulties of translation.

Even more important, however, is that

> even if we were able to look behind all these distortions and filters, we should not find what we were hoping for because the events, themselves, in their numerosity and in their details are uninteresting to the present day observer. They are without historical meaning.*

THE LINK BETWEEN THEORY AND PRACTICE

My claim in this book is simply that the world view embracing the continuity of life, the passivity of human beings, and the accuracy of history has become so fixed that as a society we are unable to let go of the

---

*Klaus Riegel's essay on dialectical psychology also focuses on the issue of history. He says, "History is always perceived as an interpreted history. In history we do not know how it really was." For example, the historical event of George Washington crossing the Delaware does not represent, in any sense, the actual crossing but represents our idea as represented in the famous picture by Emanuel Leutze (1851). This, of course, is very similar to Schama's story of the glorification of General Wolfe's death.[14]

organismic model of development long enough to consider plausible alternatives. Many fields of study can escape the impact of their findings on public policy—for example, mathematics prides itself on having no basis in reality, and therefore it should have no impact on public policy. This is, however, less true for the sciences that deal with human behavior.[15] Ideology, at least expressed as a world view or as a hypothesis, influences how we collect our data, how we interpret those data, and the results we obtain. Similarly our theories affect our public posture. That the two may very well be intertwined inextricably is a factor that social policy makers seem to have neglected. The attempt to help children often neglects the fact that the nature of the help is theory dependent. I believe that when a full discussion of the various models possible is undertaken, the connection between practice and theory and in particular between practice and the organismic model of development will become obvious.

An interesting example of the relation between theory and practice is the view of the child as a miniature adult, that development consists of the addition of more of whatever it is that the child already has and there are no transformations. This view contrasts sharply with the view expressed by such developmental theorists as Heinz Werner and Jean Piaget, who argue that an elaborate series of transformations occurs and the young child is not similar to the adult. These two views of children should have important implications for a variety of socializing behaviors. If we believe that a child is a miniature adult, as opposed to something unique, we are likely to dress children as miniature adults. Pictures of children taken one hundred fifty years ago show children in suits with top hats, ties, and shirts or in petticoats and elaborate dresses, quite similar to what their fathers and mothers wore. Now we do not consider children to be miniature adults, and we dress them differently. Although this is only a small example, it does raise the more general issue of the relation of our theories of development to our social policy.

The intricacy of the interweaving of theory and practice is exemplified by Thomas S. Kuhn's theory of the progression of science as opposed to Karl Popper's view. Whereas Popper has proposed that science progresses through the process of refutation—that is, proposed theories are rejected by data—Kuhn argues that theories rise and fall on the basis of their confrontation with anomalies, these in relation to the zeitgeist.[16] In other words, science and theories relating to truth are embedded in the general social milieu. The nature of the social milieu, in turn, will affect the theories, while the theories affect the nature of the zeitgeist.

This interaction applies particularly to theories relating to human behavior and the nature of social relationships. There can be no question that the general propositions related to the organismic model of development are not only strong beliefs found in developmental science and in psychoanalytic practice but also are strongly held by society at large. To challenge the idea that early experience affects later behavior is to challenge an idea within the science of development and, even more, is a challenge to a basic idea that we all now hold true and that underlies much of the existing social structure.

Therefore it is hardly surprising that the guiding principles behind our social policies are infrequently examined or challenged. We view our theories and models of development as axiomatic. So when we fail to raise children and produce citizens who maximize the ideas and beliefs of our culture—the ideas of freedom, of responsibility, of happiness, of productive work, and of significant interpersonal relationships—we look not to the theories that inform our social policies but to failings in how we put those theories into practice.

It is important, especially when such strategic efforts continue to be fruitless, to recognize the sweeping policy changes that could result from a change in the underlying developmental model. If, as this book attempts to show, there is much reason to question the validity of the model now in use, then such policy changes deserve to be considered.

Throughout the book, but especially in the last chapter, I focus on this problem. Indeed my premise is quite simple: that our social policy toward children and families is predicated on the organismic model of development holding that it is a continuous and goal-directed process in which earlier events, specifically very early events in infancy and early childhood, play a profound role in subsequent development. Our social policies toward families and children are designed around this premise. If, however, the alternative premise is equally likely—that there is a good deal of functional autonomy in children's development such that earlier events do not necessarily lead to or cause subsequent events—then our social policy very well may be different if we factor in the unavoidable accidents and chance encounters ignored by the organismic model, as well as the importance of the environment as it impacts directly on the child's life at that very point in time, and our social policy is subject to further transformation. In what follows I hope to demonstrate that our social policy toward children fails for the very reason that it is predicated on a rather limited view of development.

If we are to give our children the greatest opportunity for hope and happiness, we need to consider the possibility that what happens now, at any age, is most important, not what happened during infancy, and that children are active, thinking creatures who should be treated as collaborators in, not objects of, their own development. Any model of development that holds to the fixed ideas of continuity, passivity, and history as photograph needs to be questioned. We should take another look at the contextualist model of development.

Chapter 3

TRADITIONAL MODELS OF CHANGE

Is the child the father of the man? Do giant oaks from small acorns appear? Are we prisoners of our pasts, or can we, as I believe, alter fate? These questions all relate to our vision of how humans develop. While many different models of development have been suggested, and many are in current use, one in particular has captured the contemporary mind. Technically it is called the *organismic model* because the processes of development are located in each person rather than in the ongoing interaction with others and their worlds. Championed by Charles Lyell, Charles Darwin, and Sigmund Freud at the turn of the century, soon followed by Jean Piaget, it guides policy makers' strategies of social intervention and is the basis of some of psychology's best-known thera-pies. As illustrated by the following exchange I had recently with a fifty-year-old friend, it is astoundingly pervasive:

FRIEND: Michael, I'm miserable.

MICHAEL: What's the matter?

FRIEND: I'm having trouble with Susie [his second wife].

MICHAEL: What's the matter? Do you want to talk about it?

FRIEND: Not really. It's just that things aren't working out. I've always had trouble with women. I wonder what my mother did to me.

My friend's comments are not unusual. He sees his problem with his current wife—and indeed the problems with his first wife—as stemming from his relationship with his mother (who has been dead for over fifteen years), especially their relationship in the first few years of life. Most of us have come to accept that our early relationship with our parents—our mothers in particular—is one of the most determining forces in our lives. This force, like the Greek essence, resides in us and is a part of us—a trait, an enduring property that constitutes what some have called personality.[1] Some traits—or dispositions—characterize how we think, others how we feel, and still others how we are apt to behave in particular situations. Traits vary in how easily they can be altered and in how long they last. Some dispositions may exist in our DNA or in the neural network of our brains, while others, learned, can be unlearned; for example, a child's dislike for green peppers, which disappears in adolescence after the child tastes a just-picked pepper from a friend's garden.[2] My unhappy friend's complaint implied that traits formed by our relationship with our parents survive for a lifetime. He believed not only that the past had influenced his present state but also that it is likely to affect his future. Moreover, it was his early years that were particularly important.

The general proposition "Things past can affect the present" requires that we believe in history—that there was a real past, that it affected us, and that it still affects us or that there was a real past that did affect us but its effect is no more. If we believe that our past affects our present, we have to believe that there are forces that survive over time, continuing to act in the present. What is the nature of these forces? If biological, they could continue to act in some viruslike fashion. Or they could be patterns of behavior learned earlier and now firmly part of how we act—automatic, like walking. A third choice is that how we think about the past is likely to affect us in the present. For example, if you think that you were not pretty as a child, you may act "ugly" even though you are now an attractive adult.

We can understand why people behave as they do if the outcome is positive, but none of these alternatives explains why people persist in behaving in a certain way even when doing so causes them pain. Nearly sixty years ago Gordon W. Allport suggested that behaviors learned earlier can become functionally autonomous[3]—they continue despite the fact that the forces that originally produced them are no longer causing them. Such a theory only confirms our observation that it is possible to behave in a way that is not a result of the initial force. We still do not really know why things like behavior, feelings, and even desires are sustained over time.

Freud, for one, talked about neurotic repetition of behavior, suggesting that there are advantages in maintaining dysfunctional patterns, the major one being familiarity.[4] We would rather know that something will not work out well than try to change it and experience the unknown, even though the unknown may be better. Others have theorized that we become fixated at certain stages. Erik Erikson believed that if we do not solve an earlier set of problems, we cannot go on to other, more advanced problems. His life stages are a series of problems that need to be solved if we are to successfully meet the next set.[5] Others, in contrast, consider the disposition or behavioral pattern to be located in the interactions between people, sustained through the different forms of interaction that the individual maintains.[6] The disposition to behave thus is supported by the nature of the interaction, or the context. Masters, Johnson, and Kolodny, in studying sexual dysfunction, suggested that the ability to rid oneself of sexual dysfunction requires changing not only one's own habits but also the habits of others who interact with the old patterns.[7] For example, if one learned new sexually functional behaviors but continued to have sex with an individual who was party to the original dysfunction, the other's response might lead to a return to the sexual dysfunction. For this reason they suggested a change in the context, such as weekends away or a sex therapist who could serve as a surrogate sex partner.

The fact is we do not know whether any of these forces, all of them, some combination, or even yet unknown ones act on people over time. That we remain ignorant about how the past affects the present seems particularly strange given our interest in lives over time. Perhaps, because we hold to the strong belief that the past affects the present, we have not bothered to ask how this effect can come about.

Also puzzling is our attachment to primacy versus recency. Memories of yesterday's meal are usually clearer than memories of a meal eaten ten years ago, so we might expect recent events to exert more power over our behavior than those that happened long ago. The effect of recency is indeed known to play a powerful role in behavior. Yet my friend, like many of us, believes that an event that came first, his relationship with his mother, has a much greater impact on his relationship with his present wife than his first marriage, which happened in the last ten years.

I believe that what happens now or in the immediate past—something called the *context of behavior*—is more effective in controlling behavior than historical events. In contrast, most views of development incorporate the idea that events are most powerful when they occur first, even if long ago.

The theory of critical periods is a good example. A critical period is a time-bound interval having a discrete onset and offset. Before and after the period, the theory states, environmental events do not impact on future behavior; between onset and offset environmental events' effects are profound.[8] For example, if a baby duck, between twelve hours and five days after birth, is allowed to follow a moving object, the baby will forever follow that object, a phenomenon known as *imprinting*. Imprinting in animals has been likened to identification in humans since it determines whom the duck will stay near, follow, and, ultimately, mate with. The song "Mary Had a Little Lamb" tells of a lamb being imprinted on a person: "It followed her to school one day," and "Everywhere that Mary went, the lamb was sure to go!" Although this fact is not mentioned in the song, animals who become imprinted on humans are unlikely to mate with their own species.

In humans it has been suggested that there are critical periods for the development of perceptual capacities and for language development. An edited volume by Mark Bornstein presents an excellent account of many adult human behaviors thought to be affected by these critical periods.[9]

How is subsequent behavior affected by what happens during critical periods? It is believed that earlier events, when occurring during a critical time, produce or alter particular biologically based structures located in the person. But the theory that structures are changed or created to become biological-like traits may have been applied too broadly. Howard S. Hoffman,[10] working with birds, has shown that imprinting does not alter or produce structures or traits but simply causes the baby bird to be friendly to the type of bird it follows and to be fearful of all other types. Because the bird is fearful, it will follow only those birds it has been imprinted on, and thus the imprinting period—the time the bird estab-lishes its identity—appears to have a discrete onset and offset. Not so, says Hoffman, who was able to show that when he reduced the fear of the unfamiliar the baby birds would follow new types and become imprinted on them after the critical period. In other words, imprinting is not an example of a critical period; it is only an example of how early experiences can impact on later experiences and yet not be the cause of that later experience.

A simpler explanation than the critical period idea can account for the phenomenon that earlier events appear to cause later ones. Consider that a young child who learns behavior A then has more difficulty learning behavior B, not because of A's direct effect on B but because the child must first unlearn A. In our culture it takes children longer to learn bowel control (using a toilet) because they are first taught to defecate in their diapers and have to unlearn that behavior before they can learn to use the toilet. In cultures that never teach children to use diapers, they gain bowel control much earlier.[11]

In general, the idea of a critical period in human or animal development has not held up against the evidence.[12] Nevertheless, the concept of primacy is so ingrained that it lingers in the form of so-called sensitive periods—similar to critical periods but softer in tone. Although appealing in its simplicity, there is little support for the existence of a critical or sensitive period. In fact I believe there is little reason to subscribe to the traditional developmental model, in which earlier events are said to cause later ones.

There is one more point that my friend's statement addressed. He seems to believe that all of his social and emotional experiences, with a variety of people, including friends—males and females—wives, children, employers, employees, even the mail carrier, are determined by his early relationship with his mother. The importance of the mother is one of the central tenets of psychoanalytic thought that has been carried into our more contemporary thinking, appearing first in classical psychoanalytic theory and extending through the object relations attachment theory of John Bowlby. Although there now exists considerable information to indicate that fathers, siblings, grandparents, teachers, and friends, as well as mothers, play a role in our subsequent relationships, the most powerful contemporary theory of social development does not introduce these others.

The mother's role is certainly critical to any discussion of socioemotional development, but that does not mean it is as relevant in a general theory of development. This should alert us to the probability that different domains—language, social, perceptual, and emotional development—may not be best explained by any single model. The developmental process, being complex, need not be characterized, except for the rules of parsimony, by a simple model.

THE ORGANISMIC MODEL

My friend's comments about his marital life imply a set of assumptions that constitute the formal properties of the organismic model of development, enumerated below. A closer look reveals that some of them, especially the last, could in fact be irrelevant to anything but socioemotional development:

1. Development is change with a direction and therefore has an end point.
2. Earlier events are connected to later ones.
3. Change is gradual, a slowly cumulative progression.
4. Events that occur in the first few years of our lives produce the most long-lasting and powerful effects.
5. Mothers are the most important element in the child's environment and are more likely than all others to affect our socioemotional well-being, both in childhood and throughout our lives.

The first and second assumptions follow from a deceptively simple and widely held idea. My friend believes that the problems he now has with his second wife are a direct consequence of what occurred earlier in his life. "Tall oaks from little acorns grow."[13] We have accepted this idea even though nothing in my friend's experience, or that of anyone else, reveals how the process takes place.

My friend's example also suggests the third assumption: the process of development is the small accretion of an initial essence that changes by simple addition. The acorn contains all that the giant oak will be. Yet another metaphor, "The child is father of the man,"[14] suggests a discontinuous and transformational process of development. The child becomes a father—something different in essence—who in turn gives rise to another child, who in turn becomes a man. The poem does not rule out that the process may be gradual, but the issue of when the transformation from child to father actually takes place is still problematic.

Underlying both of these metaphors of growth is the idea that the past affects the present, and each represents a type of organismic model discussed later in the chapter. Which, if either, we subscribe to—whether we believe the change is gradual or sudden, continuous or discontinuous—depends on how we choose to perceive or think about the process itself. Wordsworth's child to father to man and Piaget's larva to caterpillar to butterfly (the examples often given when talking about change) are ways of thinking about discrete changes in function, structure, and capacity. The historian Everett Mendelson has argued that continuity and discontinuity are inventions of the mind. In the history of science, he states, scholars have preferred, certainly from Aristotle on, to perceive the discrete moments as a continuous distribution. For example, Aristotle said, "Things are said to be continuous whenever there is one and the same limit of both, wherein they overlap, and which they possess in common." Moreover, "Nature proceeds little by little from things lifeless to animal life, in such a way that it is impossible to determine the exact line of demarcation."[15] This idea of discrete events forming a continuum is, by Mendelson's account, a product of the way we wish to perceive the world.

Whether we perceive continuity or discontinuity in the world, however, may depend largely on our other ideas about how the world operates. For example, Western scholars have focused their attention on the smooth, accumulative transition around change, while Eastern scholars have been more impressed with the fact that, in nature, living systems always are changing and that these systems and this course of change are not necessarily dependent on what occurred previously. The idea of linearity is rejected since time is not viewed as moving in a direction. Reincarnation or repeated return as a property of life, the great circle, characterizes this view.

The Western idea of continuity embraces constancy, uniformity, seriation, and progress and, because of this, is associated with a conservative ideology. Discontinuity is linked with social and political challenge or with political radicalism. Could this explain why a developmental model embracing discontinuity gets so little attention?

That change occurs cannot be questioned; it is the models that describe it that are open to debate: "The essential model issue . . . is whether successive behavioral forms are reducible (i.e., are continuous) or irreducible, here meaning discontinuous, to prior forms."[16] The ideas of slow, gradual accumulation as well as discrete and radical change reside in ideology rather than in the data themselves.[17]

In any attempt to assess the validity of various developmental models the relation between observed manifest behavior and the underlying structures, motives, and needs must be taken into account along with underlying world views. In the study of development the Platonic question of essence versus reality takes the form of whether or not the change I see in the manifest behavior of the child is a change in any underlying structure. It is obvious that the larva and the butterfly represent very different things. However, that may have to do with surface manifestations, not with the essence of the thing. If we do not know the meaning of a thing, it is not easy to discover either what it will become or what

caused it to occur in the first place. This issue becomes one of measurement, a topic taken up in Chapter 6. As we consider the various models
of development, we need to keep in mind that change can take place in
the surface manifestations of behavior or in some basic structure or
motive leading to the behavior. Stated in another way, "continuity or
discontinuity may be concerned with the relation between the hidden
structures and competence of one period and those of another, as each
competence is embodied in different public actions."[18]

So in the final analysis we cannot prove conclusively that one model
of development is most valid. Different models have different ways of
accounting for the phenomena of change, and which one any individual
espouses depends on the person's world views. We can, however, subject
them all to a logical examination to see which one appears to hold up
best. The three major developmental models that both scientists and the
public think of when they consider how development takes place are
accretional, transformational, and what I will call *additive.* According to
the accretional model, also described as accumulative, the original process remains active. For example, physical growth continues in the same
way across a child's entire developmental range. The transformational
model relies on the idea that a second developmental process completely
replaces the first, the way the butterfly appears to replace the caterpillar.
In an additive model the first process remains active while a second
process emerges, resulting in the coexistence of both. For example, the
child can have motor knowledge while also developing symbolic knowledge. The first two models are organismic, while the last approximates a
contextual model.

An Accretional Model

The accretional or incremental model states that a particular function,
structure, or skill exists in its adult form (i.e., it will not change) at the
beginning of development. The process of development therefore involves an increase in amount rather than a change in type, though many
variations on the theme are possible. The shape of the growth is one
possibility. The form can grow rapidly in early life and then level off near
maturity, as is the case with a child's physical growth. The form also may
grow slowly at first and then suddenly take off before leveling off again.
Either way, the structure that exists at the beginning increases or decreases as a function of this process. Because the structure already exists

and changes only in amount, it is possible to view this model as continu-ous. Not all skills exist in their form at birth, however; they may appear at different points in the lifetime of an individual. The startup and increase in hormonal activity specifically related to puberty and adoles-cence constitute a prime example of developmental processes that start later in life. At a certain point after birth, on the average at the age of twelve years or so, new functions "kick in" to be followed by growth and development.

One way to think of development is as a series of maturing skills that are timed by the biology of the human species. While each of these skills may be connected—they certainly are happening to the same person—their appearance is determined by some biological program. However, as we will see when we discuss the additive model, once a skill appears it is acted on and altered by the child's adaptation to the environment. The skill is altered by each child's unique adaptive needs, so that *the skill changes but remains the same; it does not become a new skill*. For example, Noam Chomsky, the linguist, believes that language has a deep structure that exists in the biology of the child and, when maturationally ready and in interaction with the environment, results in a specific language.[19]

The world view from which accretional models derive also has implications for our parenting practices and social policy. In the case of moral behavior, we could argue based on this model that children possess the same moral sense as adults but merely have less of it. That might mean it does not have the attention-holding power in childhood that it has in adulthood, so parents probably would want to impress children's viola-tions more firmly on them by using devices designed to get them to attend to their limited moral sense and thereby make better use of what they have. Moreover, if children already have some moral sense, parental socialization may be able to produce more of it sooner. The use of punishment is an example of how adults working under this model might go about socializing moral behavior.

Think about how parents typically teach their children empathic behavior. Susie pulls Roberta's hair. Distressed by this behavior, Susie's mother wants to teach Susie what it is like to have your hair pulled, so she pulls Susie's hair. I have even seen parents bite a son or daughter who has bitten another child. These actions reveal the underlying belief that the child possesses a moral sense and that all parents need to do is remind them of it.

This view of the child as a miniature adult has been widely held. We have all seen pictures of Victorian-era children dressed as adults, a manifestation of this view of the child as a miniature adult. I am reminded of a picture in which young Tad Lincoln in top hat is standing next to his typically top-hatted father, Abe. I remember in the 1940s and early 1950s being dressed in the same type of clothes as my father; the same was true for my sister and mother. If clothes are any indication, the view of the child as a small adult gave way to the view of the child as a unique and different creature only in the middle of the twentieth century.* As the accretional model lost favor, the concept of the small adult waned, and by 1960 children already were being dressed differently from adults.

A Transformational Model

A transformational model differs from an accretional model in several ways, the primary feature being that successive behavior forms are irreducible to prior forms. Such models also have been called *stage* models of development. In these models forms are transformed through their interaction with the world. Transformation models, made most popular by Piaget, are not continuous, but most often they adhere to the view that earlier events are connected to later ones. Why else call development transformational? So for Piaget, caterpillar becomes butterfly, which becomes larva—development involves a change in structure and function. Other epistemologists besides Piaget viewed the development of intelligence as a series of transformations wherein sensorimotor ability is replaced by formal logical operations.[20] In a similar fashion, the psychoanalytic model proposed by Freud contains transformational processes.

---

*There has been a return in children's dress to something like that of adults, which may indicate a return to the idea that children are small adults. Why this has happened is unclear, but one possibility may be related to developmental research of the last thirty years. Increasingly the public has become aware that, especially in infancy and early childhood, children possess many of the same capacities and skills as adults. Studies on infants' knowledge of numbers or the ability of newborns to imitate and other research may be leading to the view that there is little difference between young children's behavior and that of older children or adults. Of course, such an idea is speculative. It rests on assumptions that clothes and the dress of children reflect, in part, adults' beliefs about child development. If we could demonstrate this to be so, the change in children's dress over the last hundred years would supply evidence for society's changing ideas about the nature of childhood and about the developmental process itself.

The child moves through a set of psychosexual stages, starting with an oral focus and moving finally to a genital focus of sexuality.[21] More recently, the object relation theorists have used a transformational model to explain how a child's early attachment relationship with his mother becomes peer friendships and then adult romantic relationships.[22] Each of these examples can be characterized by metamorphosis and change, where earlier behaviors change and ultimately assume adult forms. Even though they are transformed into entities of different form or structure, they can be connected. Thus this model features what I consider a connected process, where there is a sequence with an order and where early events are related to later ones.

The transformational model represents the prevailing view of development today, yet its underlying assumptions have been criticized:

1. The transformational model is directional. Transformations follow a particular order and direction, moving from A through B, then C, to D. Even though transformations may require the child to interact with the environment, the transformations themselves and their order appear to be relatively fixed. Yet not all children go through the same sequence. For example, while most children crawl after sitting up and before walking, not all children who walk crawl.

2. Transformations take place and therefore are not reversible: A, in becoming B, ceases to exist. This requirement implies that A, what occurred earlier, affects or causes B, what occurred later. The metaphor of the larva becoming the caterpillar implies explicitly that the larva ceases to exist when the caterpillar emerges and that there is no chance of reversibility.* This idea presents problems for the possibility of regression to earlier levels, a phenomenon that is often observed, especially under stress. Of even more concern is that, once a level emerges, only this single highest level is available for use in interaction with the environment, regardless of the task or problem at hand. The earlier levels, having been transformed, are no longer present.

3. Piaget's[23] transformational model begins with only the simplest set of motor patterns; that is, for him the developmental process starts

---

*Also an important transformational principle for Piaget (à la Hegel) is the negation of negation in which A is transformed into *not*-A without being lost. A and *not*-A are synthesized without losing A or *not*-A. Such may be possible, but within the child there does not appear to be both A and *not*-A.

with very simple behaviors that themselves give rise to all other forms, structures, and behaviors. This idea has in fact been thoroughly disproven. Tom Bower[24] showed over two decades ago that very young infants have complex sets of reflexes that appear from birth; for example, very young infants become quite upset if they experience perceptual discrepancies involving two different senses. If infants see their mothers talking to them when experimentally their mothers' voices are temporarily altered, they become upset. Like adults at a movie, where the sound track is not synchronous with the visual facial movements of the speaker, infants show recognition of these intersensory discrepant events and do so almost from the beginning of life. The list of other abilities seen too soon after birth to be readily learned, like imitation, strongly supports the idea of a complex set of abilities at the time of birth.

Relying on only the simplest of reflexes allows Piaget to take the most interactive stance since it is from this small behavior present at birth, in interaction with the environment, that all subsequent forms derive. These initial reflexes, which are part of our species's biology, are needed to start the process. While this assumption led Piaget away from a nativistic position, the presence of any unlearned structures undermines the basic transformational model.

4. Finally, the transformation of A into B requires that something be added to A for it to become B; B is different from A and, as such, is a different form. Again, this requirement is necessary if we wish to argue that A and B are different but that A and B are related and that B is derived from A. Such a view fails to satisfy logical requirements. Owen Flanagan, a philosopher of science, in analyzing the problem inherent in this view of development and of Piaget in particular, states, "If the story Piaget tells about cognitive development is right, he needs to explain how the mind builds richer and richer systems of cognitive structures." What we have is a constructivist problem: "One cannot build new and richer hypotheses out of less rich conceptual resources *simpliciter*."[25] If development is transformational, it is not clear how A becomes B; A and B are different essences, and one cannot be derived from the other.[26]

The requirements of a transformational model that insists on these principles violate much of what we know about children. One solution to this dilemma is to suggest that A and B are unconnected and unrelated. While A may participate in and be necessary for the creation of B, A is not itself transformed or lost; A is maintained as B develops—it is what I call an *additive model*.

An Additive Model

There are major differences between transformational and additive models of development. Figure 1 contrasts the two models. Like the transformational model, the additive model has directionality; it moves from A through B, then C, to D. Also as in the transformational model, development in the additive model takes place in interaction with the environment. Indeed, the environment is a very important aspect of the model. The most significant difference between the two is that in the additive model development does not occur through transformations. B may be only partially, or not at all, related to A. It may need A to come into existence, but it is not made up of A, or it may come into existence without A ever being present. Rather, B can arise as a consequence of some environmental and/or biological interaction. In this case, as the environment changes, B comes into existence. Again, B follows A but is neither of A nor caused by it.[27] Like A, B may develop further once it emerges, but transformations are not as we might have envisioned them to be. It is more like the addition of new skills and the accretion of those skills that have already emerged, for example, $A \rightarrow A_1, B \rightarrow B_1$, etc. The additive model, then, draws a picture of periods of change when new forms emerge, like B in Figure 1, followed by periods when the new form changes slowly under the pressure of adaptations with specific features of unique environments, like B_1. This model represents radical discontinui-

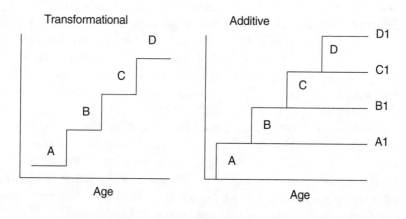

FIGURE 1.

ties and gradual changes. Such a model now exists as the best estimate of biological evolutionary change; it is called *stasis and sudden change*.

In the additive model there is no single end point, D, but rather the coexistence of all earlier abilities and skills. This allows for reversibility or regression; under stress a child who has passed the thumb-sucking stage can and does suck her thumb. It also allows for multiple use; a child who has learned to walk can still crawl if he so desires.

The existence of multiple levels allows for a set of capacities and abilities that can be employed selectively when confronted with a task; that is, the organism can choose which level to employ for which particular task. The choice of ability cannot be a function of the limitation of choice; it must be a function of some other phenomenon. Such choices are probably based on socialization factors or on a program available to the organism to choose which level to employ. Let me give an example of both.

In the first case, socialization, it may well be that certain cultural factors determine which level of operation the organism chooses. Thus, in a culture that does not use abstractions, people may be socialized to use one level to solve a problem. When, however, they are given the opportunity to use another level, they can do so quite quickly. A. R. Luria studied Russian village differences in perception and reasoning, choosing different exposures to industrialization as a means of studying socialization or contextual differences. Villagers in the unindustrialized area, when tested with problems calling for both abstraction and concrete reasoning, emphasized concrete reasoning, while villagers in the industrialized areas used more abstract reasoning. Luria assumed that the only difference between the groups was their exposure to electricity and electrical equipment as well as other forms of modern technology (this was in the 1920s). His work indicated that the level of reasoning available to the villagers was dependent on socialization since once the unindustrialized villagers received the new technology their reasoning levels changed.[28]

Individual "programming" may also account for which level is used to solve a task. If we think of these levels as involving different processes, we can recognize some levels employing different brain structures. We might suppose that people would use one level for emotional and others for nonemotional tasks.[29] As we can see, the availability of choice means that the additive model must be more contextually determined than the transformational model and that the developmental process itself cannot be understood without determining the nature of the environment and how it changes.

We should not be surprised that socialization of children differs when transformational or additive models are held instead of accretional models. Parents understand that their child does not have all capacities. For example, if the child shows little moral sense, the parent may realize that there is no parental action that is likely to strengthen the child's moral sense. Socialization practices have changed from attempts to increase the small amount of capacity to the facilitation of processes that lead later to the desired capacity. Consider the example of Susie who pulls Roberta's hair. Using a transformational or additive model, her mother recognizes that Susie is too young to have empathic behavior. Rather than pulling Susie's hair to show her what it feels like, her mother will try to prevent Susie from pulling Roberta's hair. If she cannot do that, she will indicate her displeasure, which may well lead Susie to change her behavior not so much because she has developed a better moral sense but because the negative behavior of her parents (with explanation) is an effective control of behavior.

DEVELOPMENTAL FORCES

What forces drive the developmental process itself? Where one stands in the ongoing nature-versus-nurture debate contributes to the ultimate choice of a developmental model. The most widely accepted models, be they accretional, additive, or transformational, require that the environment play a central role. In fact Piaget's desire to take environment into account was so strong that, as we have seen, he adopted a precept that undermined the very model he supported.

The Biological Imperative

Any model can contain the idea of biological forces that control the forms that exist, their sequence, and their unfolding. A biological imperative view holds that our DNA codes not only the forms or structures that we have but also the process of change. For me there is no question that a biological process as it adapts to a particular context results in the zygote differentiating and becoming, in a relatively short period, a full and complete human organism. Nor should there be any doubt that there are powerful biological processes, also in context, that result in the newborn infant's movement through the various stages and cycles of life. Even language acquisition is located in the biological processes and structures of the organism. No amount of environmental manipulation is likely to produce language from a goldfish.[30] In a similar way, the physical growth of an organism is influenced by highly likely biological processes.

Even here, however, we need to remember the role of environment in affecting development. We all know that the first generation of Japanese born in the United States were significantly taller than their siblings born in Japan. There has also been a significant height change in Japan since the end of World War II.

Biological processes also are likely to affect psychological variables. For example, there is ample evidence to indicate that consciousness, the ability to think about oneself or to think about others thinking about the self, is through maturation likely to emerge.[31] These capacities are the result of emerging biological processes. The four-year-old child's ability to take the perspective of another also is an emerging process. Thus, while the three-year-old child has trouble informing an adult about what the adult's perspective might be, the four-year-old has less trouble doing so. These kinds of shifts, although not necessarily linked in any strong way to a particular age, are the result of emerging biological processes. In a similar fashion, biological dysfunction is likely to disrupt emerging patterns and may lead to developmental delays or even failures. A child born with an injury to the cortex and surrounding tissue is likely to fall behind and may never achieve a normal pattern of development. Nevertheless, these are emerging processes that occur in a context.

While it is clear that we are all biological creatures and that no model of development dare neglect the role of emerging biological processes and genetics in how we get to be what we are, the most powerful biological process we know of is adaptation; biology is in constant interaction with and changed by the contextual features in which it occurs. We have the capacity to adapt to the most unusual of biological insults. The most recent work on the genetic and biological bases of behavior leaves little room for doubting this most simple model of change.[32] The organism's history, as well as its future, is not determined solely by the workings of its biology. For example, the damaging of structure, if the biological imperative is strong enough, should lead to functional insufficiency. Yet there is ample evidence that biology cannot account for the developmental process. The perinatal collaborative study, for example, observed thousands of children and found that none of the more than one hundred perinatal biological variables predicted the child's IQ at three and a half years of age.[33] What was predictive of the child's IQ was the educational level of the children's mothers and fathers. Such findings as these, and there are many more, indicate that, although biological processes are likely to carve out the broad species-specific functions (i.e., the functions common to all humankind), they are generally insufficient to account for differences on an individual level.

Contextual Forces

The simplest environmental model holds that exogenous factors influence the child, who is passive to their force. Behavior, whether normal or maladaptive, is primarily a function of the environmental forces acting on the organism at any point in time. In such a model the child uses the toilet and does not soil his pants because using the toilet is positively rewarded by parents and soiling pants is punished. The environment controls behavior by exerting pressure at all points in the developmental process.

Although this model may apply for some behaviors, another world view is that environmental forces act on an active child, one able to remember and learn and, most important, one capable of abstracting information from the environment so as to generate rules. Children have memories; they can think, they can plan, and they have desires. These capacities both utilize the environment and are created by it. Our hypothetical child may not soil his pants after having been punished for doing so because he remembers what will happen to him if he does. But he can learn in many other ways as well. He can imitate and learn from others' mistakes. If his mother scolds his older sister for writing on the walls of the bedroom, he learns, although he is not directly involved, that the walls should not be written on and that one who does that is likely to be punished. Our need to adapt to our environments means that children are active participants in their environments. Information may be received from the environment, but it is always actively perceived and processed. The child may be rewarded and punished, but these actions are information that the child uses to construct thoughts, plans, and values.

The role of the environment as an important aspect in interaction has been underplayed because most models of development, certainly the organismic one, seek to find the structures and change within the child. In the study of psychopathology, for example, even though we recognize that environments can cause disturbed and abnormal behavior, we prefer to treat the person—to increase coping skills or to alter specific behaviors—rather than change the environment. Yet we can imagine the difficulties that are raised when we attempt to alter specific maladaptive behaviors in environments in which such behaviors are adaptive—an exaggerated point taken by Thomas S. Szasz, who has argued it is environments that are crazy, not people.[34]

The belief that much of the force of interaction resides in the organism rather than the environment raises many problems directly related to social policy. For example, many are likely to assume that violence occurs because of individual factors, such as the XYY chromosome constellation, rather than in the interaction of the child with a particular structure of the environment. The XYY chromosome configuration was thought to represent the "super male"—aggressive, with little impulse control, and so on—and studies were done to see if prisoners were more likely to have this characteristic. The incidence of XYY in the general population was not known, however, and the entire literature blaming aggressive behavior on genetic factors was dismissed when base rates in the population were obtained.[35] Yet we fundamentally believe that people's ability to change is an attribute or trait that they possess rather than a function of the environment: if you possess the trait, you can change; if you do not, you cannot change.[36] That is the reason, for example, some people dislike overweight people, believing that they are "fat" because they do not have the will to stop eating and lose weight.

We hold fast to this position despite many observable examples of more subtle environmental control of the developmental process. In one New Jersey school district fifth graders were the "seniors" in their primary school and so were more social than the younger children, dating and going to parties. When the district altered the policy and sent fifth graders to middle school, the fourth graders became the "seniors" and as a result their social behavior changed to resemble that of the fifth graders. Such data reveal that social behavior can be influenced by the perception that one is the oldest and therefore should behave in a particular fashion quite independently of age, the trait most associated with biology.[37]

If children's behavior and their development are a function of the environment in which they live, then as long as the environment remains consistent, children's behavior should be consistent. If the environment changes, so too will children's behavior. This point of view suggests that characteristics of individuals are both established and maintained by environmental factors. This is true for normal as well as psychopathological behavior.

The environmental model of the causes of change can be readily tested, but rarely are such tests performed. This failure reflects the bias in favor of the organismic model and raises serious questions about society's commitment to change people's behavior. On the one hand, we profoundly believe that people can change, but at the same time we are less confident that the change can be brought about through interaction with the environment.[38]

Perhaps the most poignant piece of literature on the effects of the environment on people's lives is George Bernard Shaw's *Pygmalion*, a play designed to demonstrate to the upper-class English that a lower-class girl could become upper class in manners, values, and speech if given the right environmental opportunities. Shaw's environmental intervention, however, consisted of more than the three hours per day of a program like Head Start, the typical "test" of the power of context done in recent years; it was a total commitment, twenty-four hours a day, in a new environmental interaction.

One way to observe the effects of the environment on children's subsequent behavior would be to observe situations in which the environment changes. Studies of social intervention reveal interesting differences in children's social behavior. For example, infants and young children raised in day-care programs, where they interact with many different people, show less stranger fear than infants and children raised at home, alone with their families. So stranger fear, assumed to be related to maturation, appears related as much if not more to environmental differences.

The environmental model suggests that at all points in development the child's behavior is determined by interaction with the environment. Should the environment change, the child's development will change. The degree to which the environment remains consistent is the degree to which consistency will be found within the child. Invariant environments, while possible, hardly are likely. Societal structures always are in a state of change—wars, famines, floods, and disease always are with us and always lead to change. Recently we have come to appreciate that our climate can change more rapidly, in decades rather than centuries, than we had thought. Even within the family there is change. Sibling birth order effects and the fact of aging result in very different environments within a family.[39] That the environment usually is in a state of change suggests that, if continuity requires environmental consistency, we are not likely to find much. Thus, from both endogenous factors, as in the transformations themselves, and exogenous factors of changing environments, we have little support for the idea of continuity or for the idea that our fates are readily sealed. There is an equally strong argument against development as a continuous process, so our belief in the organismic model of development must rest more on faith than on fact. This being so, consideration of a contextual model is certainly warranted.

Chapter 4

DEVELOPMENT
IN CONTEXT

The organismic model of development traps us in our past. As in Freud, who believed that mental health is determined within the first six years, and John Bowlby, who believed that a mother's behavior in the first year of life is critical to all of the child's subsequent relationships, early (and sometimes very early) events are said to seal our fate. Under this model we can neither escape our past nor alter our future.

Although children change and develop, they are often viewed as complete self-contained miniature adults whose existing structures merely grow or as beings subject to relentless and irreversible metamorphosis. There is no room in the organismic model for accidents, chance encounters, randomness, consciousness, and desire. Radical discontinuities and emergent structures are rejected, and in their place stand predeterminism, progress, and gradual change. It is a model depicting passive human beings closed by their past and restricted in their future.

I believe instead that we can alter our fate. We do it every day. But why should it have taken us so long to realize this? Consider psychoanalysis. Freud's theory claimed that particular early experiences determine our future—seal our fate—except, of course, if we are psychoanalyzed. Freud and those after him said that even though early events determine our future, our destiny can be altered by later events. Thus they had it both ways: a theory relating earlier to later events in a deterministic way, and a therapy that could alter the impact of earlier events. It is strange to imagine that only a psychoanalyst could alter the past. Why not a lifetime of experiences? This illogic between theory and practice should inform us that altering fate is something we achieve every day.

The organismic model of development, most often viewed as a causally related chain of events, allows for prediction. There lies both its appeal and its downfall. Our belief in the ability to predict over relatively large spans of time has captured the interest and attention of psychologists for the last hundred years. Over that generous time span ample evidence that what happens earlier affects what happens later should have been accumulated. Yet most short- and long-term longitudinal studies have failed to find much of a relation between earlier and later events. Even when a significant relationship between variables is found over time, eighty-five to ninety percent of the association between these variables is not accounted for! Even more disappointing is that as the time between events increases, the relation between them decreases, a common finding called a *simplex pattern*. It is as if we have the power to predict the next five minutes and little beyond.

Based on the collective evidence to date—in a multitude of domains, including cognitive, social, emotional, and psychopathological—the best that can be said is that there sometimes is very limited support for the belief that earlier events are connected to later ones. We could claim that measurement is the problem—that if we could better measure the behavior over time we might be able to show greater consistency. This argument seems like a dubious refuge, however. Given that there is very little empirical evidence to support the organismic model, our strong belief in it is in fact somewhat astounding.

The organismic model, clung to out of a desire for predictability, has so far failed to predict or explain development. Now we have a choice. We can hold that this is true for measurement reasons, or we can be prepared to surrender the idea. I suggest that this organismic idea of development is only one of at least two models and that, having found the more traditional view of development wanting, we must consider alternatives.

CONTEXTUALISM

At the turn of the century, William James described a new philosophical position that came to be called *pragmatism*.[1] Within this stance he expounded a position that Stephen Pepper called *contextualism*.[2] Contextualism, for our developmental point of view, argues that to under-stand meaning we have to understand it as embedded in events occurring *now*. Contextualism is not historical; events in the past are not related to events now. James arrived at this position because for him there was no way of knowing if events in the past were related to events now.* He said, in discussing the characteristics of the mind, "The mind may change its states and its meanings at different times; may drop one conception and take up another, but the dropped conception can in no intelligible sense be said to change into its successor."[3] For James, these thoughts or properties of mind occurred in the context of the moment. As the context changed, so, too, did the thought. His pragmatic position, in which contextualism played a central role, did not utilize the concept of progress toward an end point; nor did it need the idea of a linear causal relation where earlier events are likely to cause later ones. In regard to progress and causal sequential relations, James's position is best seen as a belief that history is simply a collection of facts that are not necessarily related to one another. Such a view also questions the idea that there is an order or a sequence as an objective reality, that is, that there is something that exists independent of us, toward which we move.

We can see how different this view is from that of the early American psychologist James Mark Baldwin or that of Jean Piaget. Piaget, especially, thought of development not only as a sequence of causally related changes—that is, development as a historical theme—but as a sequence with a goal, whose order was fixed, with the child coming to this order through basic processes located in the genotype. Thus, al-though the environment was needed for the child to acquire intelligence, the sequence of acquisition and the nature of intelligence were fixed properties, independent of the child.

Because James did not accept a historical perspective or, therefore, the idea of progress, he also did not believe in an end point in the developmental process. What James did have was an interest in the self and a belief in the self as an active constructing agent. Because of this, he proposed a type of teleological theory of mind. For him the mind lent substance to our existence and was determined by our purpose. Our goals, desires, and wishes created mind, and in turn our minds created these

---

*While Pepper's metaphor for contextualism is the historical event, that is, the array or configuration of the system as it exists at a given moment in history, one instant in history need not be related to the next. For me, then, it has little historical significance.

goals, desires, and wishes. For James, then, a developmental theory would have several important features:

1. An active self exists, one capable of thinking, planning, and having goals and desires.
2. These goals and desires are best understood within a meaning system occurring now; thus the emphasis on contextualism.
3. Earlier events need not necessarily determine later events; thus there is no need to think of development as a unidirectional, bounded process.
4. Finally, there is no need to postulate progress as an essential feature of the developmental process. In other words, there is no end point in the developmental process, no final state to be achieved.

This Jamesian view, written nearly a hundred years ago, finds expression in contemporary ideas as well.[4] More recent views capture the ideas that humans have selves that play a central role in their lives and in their development. The importance of the self forces the idea of history as past events acting on the present to yield to the idea that the present reconstructs the past. That is, it suggests that our pasts are not real but a construction. In the construction, little need remain of that which led to the construction. Even more important is the idea that it is impossible ever to determine what the real thing in the past was.

This antihistorical argument has a parallel in how we now think of memory. Until recently most of us viewed memory as a photograph, an accurate representation that captured in detail all of what occurred. If our memory was so accurate, then history, too, had to be real; it had to be possible to capture the past. More recent views, however, suggest that memory is a construction that may or may not bear a strong resemblance to what occurred. Perhaps even more important, the constructed memory can, over time, undergo elaborate change and transformation. So what I remember now about something in the past may bear no resemblance to what actually occurred. If we reject the memory-as-photograph model, we need to do the same for historicism, the argument that there really is something back there in time that can be measured and that determines what occurs in the future.

Glance up from this page and look around the room you are in. No doubt you see many things. Which of them will you remember? Some would say that if memory is as accurate as a photograph, you will remember all that you have seen. On the other hand, it seems quite clear that what we perceive and what we remember will be based on our needs, either what we anticipate needing for the future or what we know we need now. In other words, memory is contextual and pragmatic, as James argued: memory or history has to do with the goals and desires we have at the point of memory. Notice that at-the-point-of-memory can be either the now when you first experience the event or any now when you remember it in the future. So, if memory depends on the meaning needed at a particular time, memory should have the capacity to alter or change, depending on the context at that point. James's proposed teleology of the mind thus makes sense; minds—or, in this case, memories—are constructed around needs, and the needs that arise are the functions of our minds.

A contextual world view also alters our sense of time. According to James, order is not inherent in nature; we create it to understand the world through science and logic. Pepper picks up on this point as well: "For the contextualist, the dimension 'time' of mechanism [the Newtonian theory of an orderly clock] is a conceptual scheme useful for the control and ordering of events, but not categorical or, in that sense, real."[5] The idea that time is relative allows us to consider an important possibility in understanding both memory and development: that history may represent not the past acting on the present but the present reconstructing the past. If we view history not as what actually occurred in the past but as a construction of what we believe occurred, we allow for the possibility that our *actual* histories have relatively little bearing on our development. Rather, current behavior is influenced by what we think our histories were. Human beings have the capacity to alter the past in light of the present.

As we can see, this backward construction of reality does not agree with our temporal sense of development as being unidirectional, going from earlier to more recent events. Essential to such a view is an active mind, a self with feelings, thoughts, and memories—the important features in determining a life course. In the organismic or passive view, events act in a unidirectional manner on people. In this contextualist view people act on and create their own lives, including their memories and their futures, through the formation in the present of future goals, desires, and needs. As Jerome Bruner has suggested, we construct a story not only to explain our past but also to explain who we are now. This story contains pieces of smaller stories, or events, which we have chosen selectively from a larger set of recollections to create the desired narrative. The events may or may not be historically correct. The narrative explains our selves as what we are, what we wish we were, or what we want to be in the future. "It is an account given by a narrator in the here and now about a protagonist bearing his (her) name who existed in the there and then."[6] This view, expounded in social psychology by Kenneth J. Gergen, also found a voice earlier in time.[7] I am reminded, for example, of the philosopher Kierkegaard's idea of existential contingency.[8] For him, fear was produced when the past did not provide meaning for the present or the future. It was the present that provided meaning to the past. A meaningful life was one in which the present was sufficient to explain the past. In other words, health, for Kierkegaard, depended on the ability to use the present to explain what we were. This demand on the present for meaning produced trembling, while what would be in the future produced fear. Kierkegaard may have been correct; we are caught between the two dilemmas.

THIS IS YOUR LIFE

Thinking about this problem, I began to explore how such a proposition about development and history might be tested. What I came up with is a sort of "This Is Your Life" experiment. As in the TV show of the same name, I imagined picking a person and then locating many of the significant people of his past. Unbeknown to the subject, I would get those people all to agree that earlier in his life the subject had behaved in a particular way, even though he had not. For example, everyone would try to convince him that as a youngster he had been very funny and loved to tell jokes. Assuming that this fabricated story was accepted as true by the subject, would this idea about the past affect his behavior in the future? That is, would he now tell more jokes or laugh more at others' jokes if he thought that the story of his past was true? If so, we would have some evidence to indicate that the fabrication had a greater effect on his future than the reality of his past. Such evidence would support the idea that what actually happened was not as relevant as what was thought to have happened.

REWRITING HISTORY

Of course, no one has carried out this study. But the work of others regarding personal memory and the role of personal narrative speaks much to the same point. I was particularly taken with the psychologist C. Lloyd Morgan's autobiography, especially given his interest in memory. He wrote, for example, that "any autobiographical sketch . . . is the story of one's self in the past read in the light of one's present self. There is much supplementary inference—often erroneous inference—wherein 'must have been' masquerades as was so."[9] Like many others now, I take for granted the view that memory of a personal event is a cognitive construction that does not necessarily bear any one-to-one correspondence with what actually happened.

This reminds me of Jean Piaget's memory of the time he and his nurse were accosted by a stranger. His family had a tradition of telling the story, and for most of his life he remembered the stranger's face. It then came as a surprise that, when his nurse was very old, she told the family she had made up the entire event.

Recently, Michael Ross reviewed the mechanisms that underlie the relations of personal histories.[10] He suggested that the first step in constructing our past involves people noting their present status; they ask themselves what they are like now and utilize this information to make a determination about the past. Ross argued that people do this because "the present is generally more salient and available than a person's earlier standing."[11] The second step in this process of reconstruction involves deciding about the likely stability of one's current self. Paying attention to one's present self is necessitated by its salience, a proposition that seems quite reasonable. The ideas embedded in this theory have much in common with my propositions that memory is a construct that may or may not reflect what actually happened if we could measure it, which we cannot, and that what we construct about our past is related to our present.

A diverse set of studies supports the proposition that our present affects our past. In one study subjects were presented with a tape recording made by a medical expert who reported that vigorous physical exercise, such as jogging, is more harmful than beneficial. A week or so prior to this message the subjects were asked to keep a record of their exercise. After the subjects received this false information, they were asked about how much exercise, in particular how much jogging, they did. The subjects' reports about how much exercise they did disagreed with the logs they had kept. Subjects exposed to the negative message altered their memory, reporting less exercise than their records revealed.

In another study Ross and his colleagues enlisted the help of university students. This time the negative message had to do with brushing their teeth. Subjects who received the negative message reported that they brush their teeth less frequently than subjects whose attitude had not been altered by the message. As Ross points out, "There is an obvious analogy between such results and the rewriting of history that occurs in [political] regimes to make past events seem more compatible with current views."[12]

If these laboratory manipulations appear unreal, there are more naturally occurring situations and behavior change to back them up. Of particular interest is a study done at the University of Michigan from 1952 to 1972.[13] This study obtained the recall by African Americans and Jews of their party affiliation during the election years of 1920, 1924, 1929, and 1932. During this period most African Americans and Jews were Republicans, because it was the progressive party, the party of Lincoln, the liberator of the slaves, and they did not become Democrats until the early 1930s and Franklin D. Roosevelt's New Deal. Being questioned about their party affiliation of thirty years earlier was a good test of whether their current affiliation would influence what they claimed had been their affiliation in the past. The vast majority surveyed recalled that for the years in question they voted Democratic. Many respondents assumed that their affiliation had remained the same over the years.

Studies on recall of substance abuse find the same kind of effect. High school students were asked to recall their use of tobacco, marijuana, and alcohol two and a half years earlier. The data again suggest that the students' current status biased their reports of their earlier behavior. Those subjects who at present used the substance reported that they used the substance two and a half years earlier, even though they might not have; subjects who reported that they did not use it at present were more likely to report that they had not used it then.[14]

Ross presented a most intriguing study of women and menstrual difficulties, suggesting that some women may inadvertently bias their recall to support the theory that they suffer extreme menstrual distress. This, of course, is not to say that they did not have menstrual distress— quite the contrary. Nevertheless, when subjects were asked to keep diaries, including information about menstrual distress, it turned out that their recall in their diaries was affected by their current menstrual distress. The recall of difficult menstrual symptoms was highly influenced by the women's current affective and physiological states. Ross's data also implied that a bias in recall may contribute to the maintenance of the exaggerated beliefs. If this is true, we have, in effect, a measure of William James's idea of mind, namely, that the mind, or memory, functions to lend substance to our existence, which itself is determined by our purpose. In other words, our belief about our current condition influences our current belief about the past, and our belief about the past in turn gives us meaning about the present.

These impressive studies from the social psychology literature support the idea that what we believe in the present affects our memories of what happened in the past. Although the study of people's recollections or memories has received relatively little scientific attention, the general finding appears to be that there is poor agreement between what happened and one's recall of what happened. More important, however, is the finding that one's present status impacts on one's recall of what was. Perhaps most relevant to our focus on development is a study done by Marian Radke Yarrow, John D. Campbell, and Roger V. Burton of both mothers' and their children's recollections of their relationship in the past.[15] In this study they gathered what they called the "baseline data," which were derived when the children were young. Through observations, tests, ratings, and reports gathered years before, information on the earlier mother–child relationships was evaluated and the participants in that research recontacted and reinterviewed. Yarrow and her colleagues found that there was little overall relation between children's recollection of their relationships with their mothers and their actual relationships with them. Mothers' recall of the earlier relationships was no better. As Yarrow and her colleagues stated, "Mothers who have had pleasant and rewarding experiences in rearing their children, mothers who feel hostile to their children, and mothers who have had especially stressful life situations may not be equally able to report on their own rearing behavior or on the behavior of their children."[16] Even more important to this discussion, however, was that Yarrow and her colleagues found mothers' and children's recall of their earlier relationships depended on their current relationships. The degree of warmth or coolness in the *current* relationship shifted the *recollection* of the past in the direction of the current status. "For groups in which the [current] relationships were rated as 'cold,' shifts in recall tended to be in an unfavorable direction; and for groups in which the relationships were rated as 'warm,' shifts in recall tended to increase the felicity of earlier times."[17]

Mothers' recollections of the preschool personalities of their children were structured so as to conform to their perceptions of the children's present personalities. For example, if the children were now seen as shy, mothers tended to recall them as having been shier in early childhood relative to the actual data collected. If, on the other hand, the children were described as outgoing in the present, they were rated as having been more outgoing when they were younger than the data suggested. This occurred not only for the dimensions of shyness and outgoingness but also for the dimensions of children's response to authority and of their independence. The shift in ratings was also true for the children themselves. If they rated themselves shier now, they also rated themselves as having been shier when they were younger.

This study of Yarrow et al. illustrates how the present affects our beliefs about the past. Earlier I suggested that recall of and belief in events in the past, whether the events occurred or not, are more likely to influence current or future events than what actually did occur. The data showed that the mothers' recall of earlier traumatic experiences, correct or not, was related to their current rating of their children's personality more than the actual measured early traumatic experiences.

THE EXAGGERATED POWER OF THE PAST

These findings have important implications for longitudinal studies. In such studies we gather data and then try to relate those data to something in the future. As mentioned earlier, the coherence among past, present, and future is most often minimal, perhaps because, in predicting the future, past events are less important than our beliefs about those events. If this is the case, then it is important to study not only what occurred in the past but also what people now believe occurred in the past. Obtaining measures on maternal behavior toward children may not, for example, enable us to predict whether or not good mothering affects children's subsequent development unless we also know what children think about their past experiences.

John Bowlby, in trying to understand the relation between children's early interaction with their parents and their subsequent development, raised the intriguing possibility that children carry with them a working model, or a memory, of their relationships with their mothers.[18] He believed that this working model of the relationship should have a correspondence with what occurred in the past but also that it might be altered by subsequent experiences. This idea obviously has much in common with the view I have been advancing, that memory is affected by current circumstances. In addition, said Bowlby, this working model affects subsequent relationships; that is, a person's model of her relationship with her mother determines her future social life. For example, a mother who has a working model of a secure attachment with her own mother is likely to behave in such ways as to establish a secure attachment with her own child. What is unknown is whether the mother's working model of her attachment relationship with her mother bears any resemblance to what actually occurred. If it does, then we can say that in this case an earlier event has affected a later one. Given what we know about memory and recall, however, it is likely that some memories of early events bear no strong relation to what actually occurred. In that case we have another example of one's belief about the past, rather than the past itself, influencing current behavior independent of what actually occurred.

To study the question of the relation among one's recollection, what actually occurred, and one's present status, I recently examined data from a longitudinal study of a hundred children followed from infancy to eighteen years of age. I wished to determine whether the young adults' perception of their own degree of attachment bore any resemblance to observations made of their early childhoods and whether their current status affected their current perception of their past. I collected attachment data taken during their infancy, data about their current lives, and, because I was interested in the models of attachment, the standard adult attachment interview they had given. In other words, I wanted to determine whether the teenagers' model of their own attachment bore a resemblance to what their attachment had been when they were infants or whether their current status affected their current model. In addition, I wanted to determine whether what occurred in their early childhood affected their current status.

As a measure of early childhood I chose the child–parent attachment relationship, measured in our laboratory when the children were one year old. I chose attachment as a representation of the earlier socioemotional relationship between child and mother because of the extensive work in this area indicating its importance as a marker of the child's adjustment. The eighteen-year-olds were interviewed about their current feelings of attachment to their parents. To get some picture of the nature of their current lives, I asked them and their teachers to fill out a commonly used scale that measures teenagers' emotional adjustment.

The findings from the three measures were quite simple. First, young adults' current attachment bore absolutely no relation to what they actually were like at one year of age, neither for the entire group of children nor even for those children who were insecurely attached earlier. I might have guessed that young adults who showed current insecure attachment models would prove to have had insecure attachments in childhood, but the results simply did not bear this out. Second, the young adults' current mental health status, as measured either by the teachers' report or by the teens themselves, bore no relation to their early attachment relationship. Here, then, is support for a general finding of discontinuity. Earlier events, at least early attachment, did not influence subsequent mental health status. I did find that approximately twenty percent of these young adults showed some mild form of psychopathology. Thus, like many studies on eighteen-year-olds, there was evidence of poor adjustment; but this adjustment was unrelated to their early attachment relationships with their mothers. In other words, there was no predictive usefulness of the attachment relationship at one year of age to that in the young adults, either in terms of their current attachment models or in terms of current adjustment. If we consider the young adults' working models of their attachment, we are forced to conclude that their working models of attachment bore no resemblance to what their actual attachment relationships were. *If attachment classification, a much-reported important characteristic of early childhood adjustment, bore no relation to young adult behavior, serious doubt is cast on the likelihood of finding data for the belief that earlier events affect later ones.*

What I did find was a relation between current life adjustment and current attachment models. Young adults who now had positive and healthy adjustment patterns had current secure attachment models, while young adults who had negative and maladjusted current lives had current insecure attachment models. Moreover, there were no complex effects, such as the past affecting current life adjustment and current life adjustment in turn affecting the current working models.

Such findings reinforce those of the Yarrow study and others like it: people's constructions of their early childhood are influenced by how they now feel about themselves, which seems quite plausible. If people are particularly unhappy at the point in time when they are asked about their working models, they are likely to describe those models in negative terms. If they currently are happy and content with themselves, they are likely to describe their working models in more positive terms.

These findings present difficulties for the studies of childhood memories. For one thing, there is no reason to believe that any memory bears a one-to-one correspondence with what actually occurred. Memories are subject to the processes involved in all representations. These include any distortions that may take place when the initial memory is formed as well as influenced by subsequent events. Some recent research on learning and memory is beginning to show how children integrate past and recent experiences and how memories are altered. What this work indicates is that memory is not fixed and can readily be affected by subsequent events.[19]

We can see the process of current experience being added to and integrated with an already existing memory at work in everyday experiences. A child remembers going to a beach when she was very young and being hit by a wave. When her parents talk about the beach, they mention that the child was wearing a red bathing suit. The child then "remembers" going to the beach in a red bathing suit and being hit by a wave. As it turns out, the child was not wearing a red bathing suit, but this does not matter since the parents' statement has been incorporated into the child's memory scheme. We now know that people's memories are capable of systematic and lawful change as a function of subsequent experience.

That subsequent experiences can affect memory has recently become a heated debate topic in regard to sexual abuse. While all the information is not yet complete, it appears that subsequent events, in this case how the child is asked about possible sexual abuse, affect whether the child "remembers" the event. A study by Goodman and Clarke-Stewart serves as a good example of this process.[20] In an experimental situation, a child is placed in a room and after a few moments sees a man enter and watches as he dusts the objects in a room, including a doll. After a few minutes, he leaves. Next, an experimenter enters and asks the child a series of questions about what just occurred, such as "What did the man do?" The child has no difficulty responding to such a question. Next comes a series of direct questions, such as "Did the man pick up and kiss the doll?" The child most often remembers correctly and answers, "No, he did not." The experimenter leaves, and another experimenter enters. This experimenter asks the child, "Did the man pick up and kiss the doll?" Surprisingly, a large number of children now report, "Yes." As more and more experimenters ask the child the same question, it becomes more and more likely that the child will answer "Yes."

We might infer that the children are responding in this way so as to be socially correct; that is, when asked, "Did something happen?" children are likely to think that maybe they should say yes and so do. But the work on sexual abuse suggests that these are not convenient answers but are more likely to be incorporated into the child's memory and therefore to be truly believed to be so.

With both life and the laboratory demonstrating that memory changes depending on the conditions that occur after the event, we are brought back to William James's contextual argument: memory, like all the other processes of the human mind, serves to supply meaning, both about the world and about the self. Meaning depends on its usefulness in the here and now or its assumed usefulness in the future.[21] Either way, meaning depends on context.

We now have support for the idea that people's working models may bear little resemblance to what actually occurred in their childhood. In fact, those models are likely to be more related to people's current status. We can see what occurred in early childhood bears little relation to what it is that people believe about their relationships with their parents; and what occurred earlier does not affect how people behave currently toward their own children. In other words, early attachment relationships bear little resemblance to what people will believe later in life or how they will behave toward their own children. If these facts are true, then the idea of development as historical reality needs to be questioned. In general, it appears that if what happened in the past has little bearing on the future, and if one's beliefs, thoughts, and recollections are based on one's current status, then the concept of development as a unidirectional bounded process in which earlier events cause later events cannot be true. Instead, we need to consider that how we view ourselves at any moment in time is important to the understanding of how we construct our lives and therefore how we influence our own development.

PERSONAL NARRATIVES AND IDENTITY

History allows us to reconstruct how life progresses, but it does not allow us to predict its progress. Because we have selves and minds, it may be difficult to show that earlier events have an impact on subsequent events. The self and its construction of reality interrupt the chain of events between past and present.

We give meaning to our behavior, both in the past and in the present. The task of the self is to construct a narrative that allows us to explain events that are occurring now. This explanation may require that we reconstruct our past to make it fit with what it is we are now, a point made by Kierkegaard in his description of existential contingency. Developmental processes serve the pragmatic function of allowing us to adapt to the present, so we might say that the end point of development is the need for meaning now. Moreover, because we are constructing organisms, we are capable of having an enduring idea about ourselves, and we have a need to find meaning that will preserve that idea.

The preservation of our identities is necessary for our adaptation. How could we exist in the world if we did not know who we are? The stories we create about our lives, our narratives, allow us to reconstruct our histories to fit with what we are now or want to be in the future and thus to preserve our identity.

Our idea of a good story, whether it be of our own life or of some other person, is one in which the pieces fit together, they touch, and one event flows into another. So we create our histories (even as historians do) by tying the actual discontinuities together to make them match our perception of human lives as continuous and directional. These life narratives also fit with our notion of causality, in that events that happen earlier affect events that happen later. Our personal life narratives must explain how we got from one point to another, so they are likely designed to eliminate discontinuities. Our narratives are, by their nature, attempts at continuity because it is our nature, at least in this age, to think of ourselves as a unity even though we may contain conflicting parts. No matter how difficult these parts may be to reconcile, in the picture we paint of ourselves all the disparate parts somehow get together and form a single me—a personality we can understand. We need to maintain our identity, and our narratives serve that need by showing how we are the same or, if we are different, how that difference came about.

Of course, it does not have to be this way. We do not have to construct a narrative that has continuity as one of its chief features. We could live with the idea that what we are now bears only a slight resemblance to what we were. If that was so, we would need a good explanation for the change. This shift in perspective about ourselves would have great impact on our notions of causality and on our notion of self. It would violate our belief that we have a history whose parts fit a linear progression.

In what way can we truly view ourselves as being the same people we were at age three anyway? We do not look, act, think, or feel like those people. It is our memory that helps us identify ourselves in those earlier individuals. How can we do this? Following Nozick, perhaps we can understand this problem if we use a rowboat rather than a person as an example.[22] Imagine we have a rowboat built of wood and that each year we replace one board of the rowboat with a new board. At the end of fifty years none of the original boards of the rowboat remain, and yet at no point in this sequence of events have we said that this is not "the same rowboat," nor, for that matter, would we think that there was not a continuous change in this boat. But, if we had replaced all of the boards of the rowboat at once, we would say that "this is not the same rowboat" and that the change was not continuous. When the parts of the rowboat were slowly replaced with new ones, what we have been calling gradual-ism, we were willing to assume a continuous process of change, a change that did not alter the identity of that rowboat. However, when we change the boards too quickly, we see that identity cannot be maintained, nor can continuity. In like fashion, people are willing to assume that the changes that occur over their fifty years are continuous and therefore do not alter their identity.

In this regard it is interesting to note that if change occurs too quickly, that is, there are too many events in a unit of time, then we are likely to experience discontinuity. Here I am reminded of at least two periods in the life cycle when this is likely to occur: adolescence and middle age, when there are many changes in a relatively short time. In adolescence the physical body changes rather quickly, and both emo-tional and psychological events also appear to undergo rapid alterations. The same is true in middle age, when we start to lose our physical abilities or our body shape changes. At such a point one of the most noticeable characteristics is the loss of identity. That is, when the changes occur very quickly, as in the rowboat, the ability to maintain identity becomes difficult. Both adolescence and middle age are characterized by rather large and sudden changes, and therefore they are associated with problems in personal identity.

Because of the pragmatics of current adaptation, people's histories are rewritten as often as necessary to maintain the idea of themselves in time. They are rewritten to give meaning to the things around them. Rather than accept the passive developmental models, which have forces acting on people through either the biology within them or the social control from without, we need a model of development that focuses on the meaning for the individual. Meaning for individuals not only speaks to how they reconstruct the past but also addresses how they are to understand how the past may or may not influence the future. Thinking, planning, active minds are capable of having desires, of creating goals, and of making plans to reach those goals. Those goals obviously undergo change. The degree to which they change is the degree to which people's behavior in the present will be altered so as to reach those goals. People are capable of altering the course and trajectory of their lives on the basis of the goals they seek to achieve, rather than on the events that occurred in the past. Indeed, people alter past events so as to provide a better opportunity for achieving their future goals.

CONTRASTING ORGANISMIC AND CONTEXTUAL MODELS

Intertwined with the organismic view of development is an idea of an absolute truth, a history that really does exist—events that really did happen, influences that really did occur. William James addresses the idea of truth and argues that truth is not a static property of something but rather happens to an idea: it becomes true; it is made true by events. History's role is to create truths. These, rather than earlier events, are likely to cause later events. People remember their pasts in the present as they find and maintain their own truth.

How, then, does this inform the problem of development? To recapitulate, the traditional model of development rests on several tenets:

1. There is progress or an end point to development.
2. Earlier events are connected to later events. I have tried to argue that, while this may be true, and while there may be some empirical data to support this position, the longitudinal data in

the last fifty years are remarkably poor in accounting for much of the variance of earlier to later events.

3. People are relatively passive to forces, both internal and external, acting on them. These forces constitute what are thought of as earlier events, and therefore it is these forces that determine subsequent events.

As I have stated, I reject this organismic model of development for a model of contextualism. Contextualism maintains:

1. There is no end point. Progress is only an idea.
2. Earlier events are unlikely to have much relation to later ones. This is especially so if the earlier events that are studied are not related to the needs and plans of the individual as they exist now or in the future. We can understand the relation between earlier and later events only if we change our more traditional view of time and argue that our current needs and desires are likely to affect what people believe was true in the past.
3. The pragmatics of current adaptation determine how people behave.

Perhaps the best way to contrast contextualism with the more traditional developmental models is to apply both to a problem in development. Consider this example. A child is being raised by a mother who is depressed. The child's condition at one year of age is influenced by her mother's psychopathology. As in most studies, we can ask, "What will that child be like when she is of school age?" Assuming that the child showed poor school adjustment, we could argue that the child's earlier adjustment pattern influenced her later development. The organismic model assumes that, in a traitlike way, the events that occurred earlier produced in the child a quality that impacted on her behavior years later. If we look at the same problem using a contextual model, we can argue that the context in which the child was raised at one year of age affected her current adjustment because there was an interaction between the child and her environment. This is a contextual finding since the child's behavior can be understood in terms of her adaptation to her depressed mother at one year. The prediction of what the child's behavior will be like at age six is not based only on her current adjustment. What is needed is to study the context of the child at six years in terms of her current relationship with the depressed mother. If the child shows poor adjustment earlier because she is adapting to the context of poor mothering, why should the child not remain in trouble if the poor mothering environment continues? The contextual model states that the child's status at *any point will be affected by the environment at that point.*

In other words, an organismic model requires us to assume that the trait of maladjustment is located in the child and that it is this trait, established earlier, that produces the later maladjusted school-age behavior. What if the mother was no longer depressed when the child was at school age? In such a case the current context would have changed and it is likely that the child would not show maladjustment at six years. As the context changes, so does adaptation.

Do early attributes, created through adaptation, cause later behavior, or is later behavior created through later adaptation? Although we recognize the importance of context in producing early effects, we fail to consider the context when we look at outcome. Using an organismic approach, we assume that earlier events cause later events, rather than testing whether or not current events are equally likely to produce the observed effects. In the few studies that have supplied data by which alternative models can be considered, the findings support the idea that current status is just as important as, if not more important than, earlier conditions.[23] In other words, developmental continuity, which we believe is located in the child, may be located in the context to which the child adapts. Nevertheless, the literature of developmental psychology is replete with examples choosing the organismic over the contextual model.

Should the context change, earlier events may have little impact on subsequent behavior. The question, then, is not how a person progresses but how the context in which an organism adapts changes over time. Rather than an orderly progression on the basis of some internally derived imperative driving the person toward an end point, it may be that contexts alter and change, sometimes in an orderly fashion, often disorderly or chaotically. It is these changing contexts that effect change in the child.

Not only will the contexts change, but our memories of them will not bear any necessary relation to what actually happened. Moreover chance and accidents, contextual in nature, are likely to radically alter any developmental progression. I take from William James the idea that, instead of progress, history is simply a collection of unrelated facts. The question, then, is not how we progress but what we are like now. What are we doing now? What comes next may be changes in context that are not predictable and not knowable before the fact. Does this mean that we, as developmental scientists, have little to do?

My analysis requires that we seriously reconsider the organismic model of development in favor of the contextual model. The contextual approach requires that we understand that behavior is produced to aid in the person's current adaptation. Such an approach reflects the pragmatic task of the person—to adapt to the current challenge. It does not rely on the past and so allows for our ability to alter our fate. The ability to think about the future, the use of our consciousness to make plans and alter past mistakes, the occurrence of chance events in the sequence of development—these are not isolated happenings but the fabric of our lives. They are, as James said, a collection of unordered facts. These factors suggest that continuity and prediction, even at a group level, are difficult and may be even more so for the individual.[24] Without an appreciation of the role of these factors in development, we will remain disappointed by our level of understanding. Albert Bandura, touching on chance encounters, has written, "Developmental theory . . . must specify [the] factors that set and alter particular life courses if it is to provide an adequate explanation of human behavior."[25] This issue, together with the work in physics and evolutionary biology that will be discussed later in this book, suggests that a developmental theory resting on the assumption that what occurs earlier in time has a direct relation to what occurs later cannot readily be supported.

Thus besides a Jamesian view of pragmatics, a Kantian view is also required, one that introduces the idea that people have conceptions of what they want and should do to reach the goals they have chosen. Each of these ideas, desires, actions, and goals can be changed. The choices are, in part, the environments that people create. Events that we like to call basic realities are occasions when "indeterminate possibilities are transformed into determinant actualities,"[26] a basic premise of quantum mechanics that needs to be applied to human life as well. A contextual approach allows us to reconstruct how life progresses but does not allow us to predict. Like historians or evolutionary theorists, our strength may be more in how we construct our narratives and less in how such narratives relate to each other over time. We need not be fixed by our pasts.

Chapter 5

PROGRESS
AND THE METAPHOR
OF DEVELOPMENT

———≈∞≈———

W hen I was a child, General Electric (GE) had a commercial that said, "Progress is our most important product." The ad intrigued me, in part because it did not make much sense to me. At the same time, I was captured by the idea. How important GE must be, I thought, if progress was its most important product.

As I got older, I learned what the word *progress* meant. I understood why a company like GE would spend large sums of money touting its virtues. Progress was as real (if not as tangible) as the latest refrigerator or range—at least in America—and it was our task to make it happen!

To this day the idea of progress permeates our lives; it exists in the way we act toward one another and in our attempts, for example, to cure sickness and disease. It exists in our belief that we can become better people—more moral or more psychologically healthy. We believe that progress is the way the world is and always was, the way things are meant to be, and the thing we should all strive for.

Admittedly, it seems almost silly to question whether progress is "the way of the world." Does not everything living progress? Flowers grow; they progress. Children get big; they progress. Adults get better at tennis or skiing; they progress. Then again, it is hard to consider progress part of the human condition when we inevitably confront old age. How is it progress to get sick, lose vigor, become forgetful, and die? Despite undeniable signs that change does not always take that direction toward the better and that our commitment to progress does not always serve us well, we hold to our belief in the organismic model of development, which rests on the concept of progress. Because the tenet of progress impacts so strongly on our notion of how to facilitate human development and thus informs our social policy and child-rearing practices, we are obligated to scrutinize its validity and that of the organismic model of development. What exactly is progress, and what is its relationship to development? What benefits might accrue to our society if we dared propose that change is characterized not so much by progress as by adaptation?

A UTOPIAN IDEA

Progress is obviously a type of change. But while change implies only difference, *progress implies change in a particular direction*. If there is progress, there must be a set of events in a sequence—some elements occurring earlier and some later—with the sequence having direction and that direction leading to an end point or goal. Inherent in the term *progress* is the idea that the goal is both valuable and possibly achievable. In other words, to hold up the idea of progress is to claim, "Things can get better." But can they? Do they? Should we expect them to?*

The idea of progress is a utopian belief, and it flourished at the beginning of this century, flowing from the ideas of gradualism and of earlier events being connected to later ones proposed by Sigmund Freud in psychiatry and Jean Piaget in cognitive development. Both saw change as having a direction toward a goal, and both thought that goal achievable, a birthright of humankind. Freud embraced the idea of progress as it relates to psychological development and mental health. Psychoanalysis had us believe that a perfect childhood was attainable, and if it failed to materialize, we could solve our early problems later, through therapy. Piaget also embraced the idea of progress, accepting as truth the idea of stages and of transformations of earlier structures, all leading to an end point or goal: logical mathematical reasoning found in what he called

---

*Ford and Lerner have talked about successive change, a kind of probabilistic directionality that avoids teleology. I think such a view unlikely, but a possibility nevertheless.[1]

formal operations. In the natural sciences the optimistic belief was held that it was possible to know exactly how the world was put together—there was an end to knowledge. We had also seen progress in the products of the Industrial Revolution. Meanwhile, President Woodrow Wilson fought World War I to "end all wars." Even the way war was to be waged supposedly reflected progress. According to the Hague and Geneva conventions, civilians were no longer to be targets, combatants were to be treated more humanely, and even prisoners were seen as deserving the basic necessities.

By 1930, however, almost all agreed that "the hope of some vital state of earthly perfection . . . is the deadest of dead ideas, . . . one notion that has been thoroughly blasted by the facts of Twentieth Century experience."[2] The barbarism of the Nazi and fascist period shattered our belief in progress as related to the goodness of people. Sadly, more recent geopolitical events have demonstrated that the period from 1914 to 1945 was no aberration or quirk in the history of human behavior.

We may no longer aspire to a utopian society or the moral perfection of the entire human race, but we continue to cling to the idea of progress, perhaps because we've been doing so since it was first introduced in the West by Christianity.* Progress, as implied by the idea of a life hereafter as a higher state than this earthly life, was not a component of religion for the Greeks or the Romans after them. Although both had a heaven and a hell, the people did not achieve these states through any behavior of their own. The gods might mate with human beings and produce demigods, they might become angry with or wish to protect a warrior or king, but there was no clear progress that a mortal could aspire to, either becoming a god or behaving in such a way so as to live on Mount Olympus with the gods.

While Judaism brought a monotheistic element into Western religion, progress still was not a major theme. Heaven and hell were undeveloped themes made more real and concrete only as Judaism was exposed to the redemptive idea of early Christianity.

This is best seen in the story of Job, which consists of an old version to which a relatively new ending has been added. When God is asked why Job, who lives a just life, has been punished and lost his family and

---

* I am indebted to Christopher Lasch for his excellent account of the topic.

friends, his wealth, and his health, God responds: Who art thou to know of God's will?

> Who is this that darkeneth counsel by words without knowledge?
> . . . Where wast thou when I laid the foundations of the earth? . . .
> Has thou commanded the morning . . . ? Have the gates of death
> been opened unto thee? . . . Doth the eagle mount up at thy com-
> mand . . . ? Shall he that contendeth with the Almighty instruct
> him?[3]

The original story is meant to inform us that there may be no reward for one's actions. If a man as good and just as Job is severely punished by God, what chance does anyone have who lives a "proper" life? Such a harsh story, containing no progress in either this world or the next, was ultimately deemed intolerable, so under the influence of early (pre-Chris-tian) messianic and Hellenistic ideas the story of Job was given a new ending: Job's actions are rewarded by God, and thus redemption is possible, at least in this life. Judaism is based on action in this world. Deuteronomy is filled with a code for human behavior in which God's blessing is implicit but the outcome of that blessing is unclear.

Early Christianity, on the other hand promised a better life in the hereafter as the redemptive consequence of living a just life now. What was important was not how one lived now but what would happen in the future—a clear promise of progress.

The Precarious Balance of Hope and Despair

Progress is appealing to all of us, because it allows us to bear suffering in the present knowing that the future will be better. The possibility of progress gives us hope.* Each of us has pain and disappointments, but hoping that they will disappear enables us to endure, and thus hope is terribly important to us. Interestingly, while hope rests on the belief that things can get better, it makes no inherent assumption that there is an order to "getting better."

Whether it is the emotion of hope or the idea of progress, we take it

---

*Hope and progress are similar, but I prefer to see hope as an emotion, a feeling, while progress is an idea. See Martin Seligman's book Learned Optimism for a full discussion of the importance of hope in everyday life.[4]

for granted, assume it is good, and focus on how to achieve it. We equate the belief that progress is possible with an optimistic and active, rather than proactive, stance. This belief allows us to act. It moves us to try harder and to improve ourselves, others, and the society in which we live. Many of us believe that in a democracy an individual can make a difference; all we need to do is work hard—forming interest groups, getting people to vote in elections, getting information out, and picketing—to make a more just society. There are, however, others who do not believe that any progress is possible. They say that all politicians are the same and that it makes no difference what we do since it will turn out the same anyway.

The belief in progress can have important negative implications as well. We often end up disappointed, disillusioned, and profoundly dissatisfied over the facts of our lives. Whatever progress we make, there still is more progress that we could achieve. Having denied, for the most part, the religious idea of progress—the idea that we can endure any amount of suffering now for a good hereafter—we continually are confronted with the fact that there is, in fact, no end point to progress. After all, how smart is sufficiently smart, how rich is sufficiently rich, how kind is sufficiently kind? In *The True and Only Heaven: Progress and Its Critics*, Christopher Lasch describes how the idea of unending progress also is captured by our economic system. He tells of a Massachusetts bookbinder who, in 1870, said, "As people are elevated and improved in body and mind, the wants of body and mind are multiplied. On this simple fact depends all trade, prosperity, and wealth."[5] So the quest for progress results not only in present dissatisfaction but also in more wants of both mind and body, which lead to even more desire and failure.

Because there is no end to progress, we always are in a state of searching for, of becoming, never of being. It is not the present that is the end point but some undefined state, one that we never will reach, although we always will hope for it. The idea of progress, then, brings discontent with the present. One consequence of this dissatisfaction may be a turning toward the past or toward nostalgia.* If the future is not rich with possibilities, if our goals and desires continue to multiply as we

---

*Some people continue, even in the face of failure, a never-ending search for progress. These people are the saints among us, and we must always be thankful for their idealism in spite of all they know about the world in which they live.

achieve them, there may be only the idealized past to sustain us. "For those nourished on the gospel of progress, idealization of the past appears to exhaust the alternatives to a tiresome and increasingly unconvincing idealization of the future." Lasch goes on to say, "Just as we should reject the thoughtless equation of progress and hope, so we need to distinguish between nostalgia and the reassuring memory of happy times which serve to link the present to the past and to provide a sense of continuity."[6] Our nostalgia about our histories is necessitated by our disappointment in progress. So the idea of progress is a double-edged sword, on the one hand bringing hope and on the other despair.

THE IMPOSITION OF PROGRESS ON DEVELOPMENT

When we impose the idea of progress on human development, we are taking the teleological approach of assuming that things in nature are directed toward some end or purpose, in this case equating a child's maturation with the child's "getting better" or becoming perfected. But the existence of such an end point raises several problems. First, it raises the obvious question: What is the goal? If we cannot define the end point, then we do not know toward what the child is supposedly progressing and the concept of progress in this context becomes meaningless. For Piaget the end point of thought was the ability to think in abstractions, a mathematical–logical way of viewing the world. For Freud it was the genital phase of sexual development, the ability to seek sexual pleasure through genital stimulation. Piaget's analysis does not allow for the newest way of thinking about the universe, since his system was based on a Newtonian view of the world, while Erik Erikson's life stages suggest that psychosocial development has no end point. From a practical point of view, contemporary research on development uses very different end points to predict toward. Some studies focus on the causes of the end point of language acquisition at the age of two, others with the end point being grade school entrance ability, others high school attendance, and still others success at parenting. While few studies have looked at the causes of adjustment to old age, I am sure this end point too will be considered.

Second, who determines that goal? The existence of a goal implies something predetermined for us. It could be located in the gene pool or in the social structure of the environment, but in either case it (whatever the *it* is) causes the progress and has "in mind" an end point. It is a limited system. But the idea of progress, at least in modern times, implies freedom, the ability of the person to achieve all there is to be had. If progress involves a set progression, it implies a built-in limitation, but in contemporary society we believe that we can achieve anything we set our minds to. Thus, progress has the meanings of both restriction and possibility. What progress has to mean in a logical sense and its use in the common sense should alert us to the complex nature of this concept and the need to examine its validity.

Third, the existence of a developmental end point suggests that one path will be better than the others, either because that path will be more likely to lead us to our goal or because it will take us there faster. As an end point, obviously any goal must be the end point of a certain path. Also, the number of paths that lead to a particular goal must be limited since all paths cannot possibly lead to the same goal. If they did, there would be no connection, no developmental sequence, and therefore no prediction. Certainly this would not satisfy the organismic model. But even the possibility of a limited number of paths leaves us with the question of how many there might be and whether all of them are equally good. So we are faced with the conclusion that any end point, or goal, must be reachable by a single best path.

This concept of progress leads scientists to devote too much time to finding that one path—a fruitless endeavor since it cannot take into account accidents, chance encounters, and consciousness. The best path idea also threatens to make us insensitive to individual differences and leads us to develop single programs of intervention for all children—the standardized curriculum of school or of child-rearing techniques.

If we look at the process of development over the entire human life span, it is difficult to state not only what the final *desirable* end point is (assuming death is undesirable) but also what the various goals along the way might be and how they are associated with one another. Walking early is unrelated to reading ability later, and the goals of development continue to change, from getting the child to speak, to seeing that she reads, to ensuring that she does well in college, to seeing that she raises bright children, to seeing that she retains her memory in old age.

Probably most alarming, however, are the sweeping consequences of viewing children as always becoming, of never being at a point that in itself is good but only possibly on a path to the good. On this basis a child's play behavior is not likely to be considered good just because play itself is good but because play leads to creativity or some other goal. If it could be shown that children's play does not lead to more creative problem solving or to greater cognitive capacity, we might not be prepared to allow children's play because we have not been able to articulate a model of play as play that has any value of its own.

If this possibility seems far-fetched, an examination of many social intervention strategies reveals that it has certainly appeared in practice. Many years ago I was asked to serve as a consultant for a project that had as its central thesis the idea that if children's diets were improved they would do better in school. Notice that the idea of a better diet was linked not to the goal of proper nurturance but to the goal of better school performance. To test this idea, the investigators educated poor mothers on nutrition and what kinds of foods they should have in the refrigerator. Many months and a great deal of money and energy were spent on teaching mothers how and what to feed their children. At the end of a year it was found that mothers had significantly altered the kinds of food they had in their refrigerators. Soda had given way to milk, potato chips to bread without a lot of preservatives. Mothers had learned to change their children's diet. The study, however, was deemed a failure because the children did not do better in school. Although their diets had changed, this change did not result in better school performance, and since school performance was the end point, the study had failed!

CHANGE AS ADAPTATION

Although Freud and Piaget saw development as a progression, one where immature structures and processes moved toward more mature ones, the idea of progress was not found in the writings of all nineteenth- and twentieth-century thinkers. In fact, Charles Darwin's theory of species development was antithetical to the idea of progress. As you recall, his theory of evolution rests on the principles of random mutation to produce change and adaptation to determine whether such change will survive. That is why Darwin's view of evolution was and continues to be so vigorously resisted and why it was considered such a dangerous idea. Progress, as concept, requires not only that there be a direction to change and that change move toward an end point but, perhaps more important, that some underlying mechanism bring this about. In the European mind, in general, that mechanism was God's will. Progress implied order and direction, and that order resided in the mind of God. Then along came Darwin to lay waste to this aspect of evolutionary theory. By arguing in the first place for the principle of random mutation and in the second place for the survival of those mutations on the basis of whether or not they increase the adaptive likelihood that the individual or species will survive, Darwin did away with God and progress. Darwin's theory of the evolution of life was totally irreconcilable with the idea of progress or order established outside the system that is changing.

Although Darwin avoided the problem of progress, arguing instead for the idea of natural selection or adaptation of the species to its current environment as the major force of change, many of those who followed him saw in the idea of evolution another source of progress. God was replaced by the idea of the survival of the fittest and with it the idea of social Darwinism. Nature, instead of God, became the force behind change, and change again became the idea of progress.

Unfortunately, Darwin's great discovery also contained an assumption that was unwarranted and that his friend T. H. Huxley warned him against. Darwin's theory of natural selection consisted of random change—changes that had no purpose or plan—and adaptation: changes that survived to the degree to which such changes are adaptive to current conditions. While these two ideas remain his greatest insight, Darwin also believed in gradualism: the idea of slow and continuous change. He stated that nature "does not make sudden leaps" but proceeds gradually. It was this idea that Huxley warned him about and that has been shown to be questionable. Darwin's gradualism more than the other two points is what is often remembered and places him beside Freud and Piaget in regard to the idea of development, in particular the organismic model of development. Interestingly, Darwin's two main points, random change and current adaptation, place him more in line with William James's contextual model. A little bit of Darwin for each model!

Although the evolutionary position of Darwin warned against the idea of progress because of the teleological errors inherent in the view, the more commonly shared view still is that there is progress when the single-celled organism evolves into more complex organisms, such as humans. Natural selection does not argue for progress. It is hard to imagine why amoebas or, for that matter, a large colony of ants would be less progressed than human beings. No distinction based on progress should be made between ants and human beings since each group has adapted to its unique environment. As Darwin pointed out, adaptation to current context and random change, rather than progress, should be the important considerations in biological development. Although this is well known, we often fall into the teleological trap when we think of evolution as progress. It is the trap that leads to the notion that humans are made in God's image and that evolutionary processes moved in this direction.

Within the study of human development the source of progress is believed to be in the child's experiences or genes or both. It is a set of biological rather than moral factors that leads to progress. Through virtue we become morally better, and in development the transformations and structures become more complex. In both cases change is seen as progress.

Piaget, like the structuralists before him,[7] was interested in exploring how children think and so gathered a large body of information across a variety of tasks to explore differences in thinking. Finding that children tended to think differently from some adults, he concluded that there is a sequence, invariant and biological in nature, in which certain kinds of thoughts develop. Those labeled of a higher order were so designated for a variety of logical reasons, but Piaget also claimed that they were of a higher order simply by virtue of coming later. For Piaget, as for many others, abstract reasoning and formal operations are higher levels, not just changes from concrete operations or sensory motor operations. Developmental theorists like Heinz Werner, who take a broad biological perspective, also see development leading to higher order capacities. In particular, development is seen as increased differentiation and complexity, as well as transformation from one level to another. This movement toward a higher order level is in fact what is meant by development.

Although Piaget has not been seriously challenged on the idea of progress in thinking, his idea concerning different levels of thinking about moral reasoning has come under particular attack, most notably by Carol Gilligan,[8] who has pointed out that different ways of thinking about moral dilemmas do not imply that one is better or higher than another. One does not necessarily progress from "lower to higher" order in moral development. There are different ways, not necessarily better ways, of thinking. The same problem occurs when we compare different groups of people or when we look at differences between children and adults.

Similarly, human ontogeny reflects change, not necessarily progress. When nonindustrialized people fail to show formal operational thought, they often are considered to think as young children rather than different adults. This anthropological classification of different peoples on the basis of some believed-to-be-fixed and progressive pattern of thought obviously leads to horrendous ideas about the nature of adults of different cultures. A. R. Luria and Lev Vygotsky, in a now-classic study,[9] found that adult peasants' thinking was influenced by the nature of their techno-logical environment. Adult thinking, characterized by formal operations, existed in those peasants exposed to modern schooling and technology, whereas different mental capacity was shown for those peasants without such environments. Luria and Vygotsky argued that ways of thinking were influenced by the nature of the environment in which adults found themselves, not limited to some *progressive* sequence with an implied higher or better level.

Phylogeny, ontogeny, and cross-cultural findings imply change. Pro-gress should be thought of as a sociopolitical and religious doctrine, but it can be understood only in the context of adaptation, not in terms of some absolute moral or biological principle. Unlike the organismic, the contextual model of development does not need the idea of progress.

I believe that to understand the nature of development and how our ideas about development influence child-rearing and social policy prac-tices, we must recognize the dangers inherent in the concept of progress. This recognition allows us

• *First, to perceive the child's behavior as uniquely different, important in its own right, independent of what it will lead to.* The child is not a miniature adult but a child, with childlike needs, feelings, and desires. Children's play is good because it makes them happy and social now, not because it makes them better adults.

• *Second, to be more tolerant toward others, coinhabitants of the society in which we live, whose differences can be viewed as differences rather than inadequacies.* The elimination of progress denies to the argument of individual difference any moral tone. Difference is just that, neither better nor worse. The consequence of such a view is the redistribution of services, including types of school and money spent for students less on the basis of perceived innate inadequacies and more on the basis of need or adaptation.

Dislodging progress from its central position in the metaphor of development also relieves us of a burden that has vexed thinkers for millennia: the attempt to predict from earlier events or stages what is likely to happen later. If it were not for the idea that progress underlies change, there would be no attempt to construct a predictive science of development. The research findings that earlier events do not predict well later ones, the overwhelming conclusion of nearly five hundred years of research on human development, should cause us little concern as long as we focus our efforts on explanation. Evolutionary biology does not require prediction but rests on its power to explain. This is a sufficient goal for a scientific endeavor. Surrendering the idea of prediction as the sine qua non of a mature science frees us to turn our attention to more complex models of change as discussed in theories of catastrophe or complexity and to be prepared to understand that accidents, unplanned events, and self-determination are important factors in the development of species, nations, groups, families, and individuals.*

It is difficult to surrender the idea of progress, perhaps nowhere more so than in the United States, where the idea of progress and the metaphor of development are held high. Our very ideology and nature speak to the idea of endless possibilities, the desire for life, liberty, and the pursuit of happiness. But we must dare propose that change is characterized not by progress but by adaptation.

---

*Even so, the mind often rebels at the idea that development is a random event. How could it be the case that a flower randomly arrives at a shape or smells in a given way, given the myriad possibilities? More important, how could a single fertilized cell differentiate itself in an orderly change that after nine months results in the birth of the human child? Even more impressive is how in all the changes that take place in nine months going from a fertilized egg to a human being, there are so few dysfunctions in most newborn infants. The simple trial-and-error idea that all of this came about randomly is difficult to believe. While it is true that it is possible to get thirteen spades in a hand of bridge, the likelihood of that is quite low. One way to understand this conundrum is by examining the theories now being evolved about chaos and in particular the theories about complexity.[10] Complexity theory utilizes the idea of random occurrence and adaptation to demonstrate how complex structures arise without the need to evoke either the idea of progress or the idea of predetermined genetic coding. Complexity, like any theory of change, is not predictive in nature.

Chapter 6

BEHAVIOR SERVES
MANY MASTERS

From ancient runes to the Mona Lisa's smile to the crying of a woman, human beings have spent much time trying to unravel the enigma of human behavior. Does what we see or hear have meaning, and if so, what is it? Largely our efforts to find out have gone unrewarded. Even when runic carvings are translated into modern English, do we really know what fifth-century Anglo-Saxons meant by those words? Will we ever know what Mona Lisa meant by that smile—or, for that matter, what Leonardi da Vinci intended? Despite the worthy efforts of Deborah Tannen[1] and others, will men and women ever understand each other?

Throughout history people have been aware that things are not always as they seem, that the way a person acts does not always tell us what that behavior means. It is surprising then that the science of development relies so heavily on studying manifest behavior at one time as it is related to manifest behavior at another time. Psychologists, of course, do attempt to discover the meaning of behavior in their work and recognize that behavior serves many masters. But adherence to the organismic model forces many to try to infer continuity from behavioral observations, a goal not yet reached. Rather than reject the organismic model, some psychologists have responded by concentrating on methodology and measurement issues. It has been widely held that if we only could find the proper measurement instrument, we could show that earlier events cause later ones.

When thirty years ago I wrote a paper titled "The Meaning of a Response, or Why Researchers in Infant Behavior Should Be Oriental Metaphysicians," I too thought that the failure to demonstrate continuity could be attributed to a variety of factors concerning the measurement of behavior.[2] Besides not having measures of behavior that referenced the essence of the construct that we wanted to study, such as intelligence or attachment, we also were faced with the changing meaning of behavior, how attributions about behavior differed for different people, and, finally, that behavior had different meaning depending on its relation to other behavior. I now doubt that these problems can be solved through improved measurement.[3] I believe, in fact, that the dilemma of essence (meaning) versus reality (overt behavior) makes it impossible to show continuity or predictability in development. What is likely to be more revealing is observation of behavior-in-context.

In the Osteria Botecia Lornano, in the Italian hamlet Lornano, I sit and watch the other diners as my waiter approaches. He speaks no English and I little Italian, so what he says to me I cannot understand if we mean by *understand* that I know the meaning of the sentences he utters. What I do know is the context of those utterances. He does not ask me my shoe size, which he might if I were in a shoe store. He asks me what I would like to eat since minutes before he has brought me a menu. I understand what he says, which is, loosely, "What is your pleasure?" since in this context he, the waiter, and I, the patron, share meaning.

Behavior has little meaning in itself but derives its meaning only from the context—the relation of the behavior of the child to other behaviors of the child, the relation of the behavior of the child to another's behavior, or the relation of the behavior of the child at one point in time to the child's behavior at another point in time. In our attempt to understand the development of the child, it is the last context that is most often used to infer meaning; that is, the observation of the same behavior over time or different behaviors over time is likely to inform us about change. While it is difficult to infer meaning from behavior even in the context of other behaviors, the task of inferring meaning by observing behavior—either the same or different ones—over time and different contexts is nearly impossible. It is this problem that makes the study of development difficult.

Even more problematic, however, is the question "Whose meaning are we talking about?" Is it the meaning assigned by the child through the child's behavior and the behavior of others? Is it the meaning of the parent or the meaning the parent assigns to the child? Or, even more remote, is it the meaning assigned by the scientist to the child's behavior? Meaning must be understood not only as the relation among things but also as an interface among other people assigning meaning. Richard A. Shweder, a cultural anthropologist, gives a vivid account of the possibility of multiple, as well as real, meaning systems and shows how the meaning system assigned by one person or one culture to a set of perceived coherent behaviors may be very different from and just as real as the meaning system assigned by others.[4]

It is easy to see how this can occur in a study of development. If we wish to see continuity across time or across development, we can assign the same meaning to a similar event: the smile of a baby and the smile of an adult could be assigned the meaning of happiness. Or, if we choose, we can assign the same meaning to different behaviors because of our belief that the same essence underlies the production of both behaviors: the cry of a baby is an active attempt to overcome a frustration, while for the adult the behavior reflecting the same processes is task persistence.

The problem is that any assignment of meaning is related to one's world view. Those who believe in the continuity of development, in the gradual accumulation of skill or capacity, are apt to assign similar meaning to one behavior over time: the cry of the baby represents the same thing as the cry of the adult. Where this kind of thinking can lead us has been seen many times. In the not-too-distant past, for example, we believed that children do not suffer from depression simply because the behaviors that mark depression in adults did not appear in children. Those who think of development as containing discrete changes, in contrast, would assign different meaning to the same behavior over time: the cry of the baby represents an attempt to overcome frustration, while the cry of the adult represents hopelessness.

This latter view seems sensible, but does it allow any predictability? I have argued in the past that behaviors do change their meaning over age and that these changes come about through maturational or social pressures—that behavior meaning changes in predictable ways. Now I am no longer sure that they do since it is not clear how we are to know in any a priori way which behaviors at an earlier point in time are likely to go with which behaviors at a later point.

THE RELATION BETWEEN THE ESSENCE
AND THE REALITY OF BEHAVIOR

For the most part human behavior is a symbol system. It does not necessarily bear a close representation to the thing it makes reference to. Our behavior could have evolved so that the pulling of an earlobe meant "Yes, I want to have lunch," but instead we have evolved an abstract symbolic system. When someone asks if you are interested in having lunch, you might respond with yes but in fact mean no or might in fact say no when you mean yes. It would be impossible from this symbol system to know exactly what was in your mind. You might not even know yourself what is in your own head. We often do not say what we mean. At a dinner party the other night, I was served a barely edible meal, yet when I was taking my leave and was asked, "I hope you enjoyed the dinner?" I said yes when in fact I really thought no.

Even without language, we can observe the discrepancy between behavior and meaning. If I smiled at a joke you told, you would probably believe that I was amused when in fact I might not have been; I may only have behaved as if I were. We all mask our inner state by manipulating the neuromusculature of the face—children learn how to mask their expressions by the age of two or three[5]—making it very difficult for any observer to understand manifest behavior.

Yet it is the meaning of behavior—its relation to the process or construct that it is used to index—not its physical characteristics, that reveals something about development. If we assume that a given construct or process is stable or continuous over development, must we assume that the behavior we measure in any situation also is stable? Clearly not. Moreover, if the behaviors at the two observation points are the same, are we any more justified in concluding that the underlying construct has remained stable?

How do we know if the same behavior serves many masters or different behaviors serve the same master? Since continuity requires either stability of the same behavior over time or stability of different behaviors over time, this problem is central to the question of whether earlier events are related to later ones.

In *homeotypic continuity*, also termed *phenotypic* or *isomorphic continuity*,[6] the behavior remains stable or consistent but the meaning behind the behavior changes. The same behavior serves many masters.

Suppose we observe that a one-year-old child stays near her mother when the mother and child are in a strange room. Staying near could be assumed to represent the construct of the child's need for comfort. One year later, when the girl is two years old, we repeat our observation and find, again, that the child stays near her mother in a strange room. At this age, however, staying near could represent the construct of the desire to play with her mother rather than to find comfort.

In *heterotypic continuity*, also called *genotypic* or *metamorphic continuity*, the underlying construct remains the same, but the behavioral expression of that construct has changed. For example, in a study of mine, children at very young ages (two months) learned to pull a string to turn on a picture. After they learned to do this, they were then frustrated by having the apparatus fixed so that pulling the string did not turn on the picture. The infants showed two different sets of behavior. Most showed an angry face and vigorous increases in their arm-pulling behavior. Others showed sad faces, cried, and stopped pulling the string. These two sets of behaviors were taken to represent the underlying structure of anger on the one hand and sadness on the other.

What we wanted to know was whether an angry child remained angry over time, so we asked the mothers of the infants to bring them into the laboratory with their favorite toy, and we observed them again, at the age of eighteen months. We took the child's toy and put it under a Plexiglas box, asking the child to get the toy out. What we found was not a consistency of behavior over time but a transformation in behavior. The children who at two months had shown anger at being frustrated now at eighteen months spent more constructive time trying to get the toy out of the box. They were not angry; they were persistent.[7] The children who had shown sadness now showed little persistence. Different behaviors served the same master.

Stability of behavior most often is used to infer continuity of construct if, for example, there is a high correlation between behavior A at time 1 and behavior A at time 2 or if there is a high correlation between behavior A at time 1 and behavior B at time 2. This method of inference, however, is flawed. Stability means that in a group of children each child maintains her ranking either on the same measure or on two different measures over time. In the case of a single measure we could look at the height of Felicia, Cloris, and Jennifer at one year. If Felicia is the tallest and Jennifer the shortest and this remains so at a later age, we say that height is stable. Correlational analysis comparing the order at each age is used to determine stability. But stability as indicated by a correlation between behavior A at one age and behavior B at another has unclear implications. In this case what we call stability does not necessarily imply continuity.

Our findings with the infants showed that heterotypic continuity could not be demonstrated until we were able to understand the meaning of the early behavior as it related to the new behavior. We had thought that the angry face and increased arm pull had represented the underlying construct of anger, but finding a subsequent relation to persistence required us to redefine the meaning of the earlier set of behaviors. The meaning of the earlier set of behaviors was not anger in the sense of aggression or violence but the anger associated with will or the attempt to overcome frustration. It is the type of anger that leads us to persist. Our belief in the meaning of the underlying construct of anger that we saw at two months was changed by its association with other responses later in development. We could not predict from an earlier point what the response would be later. Continuity could be established only in a post hoc fashion.

What behavior means is particularly difficult to determine for any organism undergoing rapid change, such as a child. The search for consistency in behavior meaning becomes a formidable task when the organism starts out with relatively few, undifferentiated behaviors—an infant, for example—and those behaviors become through development considerably differentiated over time. An infant tends to stay physically close to one with whom he has a close and secure relationship. An adult in a similar relationship is likely to maintain contact through a variety of means, not just by staying close but also by writing, calling, and thinking about the person, among other means of contact maintenance. Even though the underlying structure of love or secure attachment exists in both cases, the behaviors that serve it, physical closeness and mental elaboration and representation, differ.

One set of factors that influences behavioral expression is socialization. The effects of socialization, in part, are the alteration or creation of behavior, and it may be that socialization acts to change the meaning of behavior as a function of developmental level, situation, or cultural demand. With increased age and as a function of gender and of cultural demands, crying, for example, becomes a less socially acceptable behavior. Therefore the meaning assigned to it by adult caregivers—and consequently their response to it—changes. In turn how the child uses crying as a form of expression is likely to change.

Finally, one of the most obvious difficulties with trying to understand the meaning of behavior is that the task requires generalizing, which means removing the behavior from the unique context in which it was observed. Without that context, does the behavior have any meaning at all? Can all the minute details of place, time, and circumstances be sorted to yield an abstract behavioral pattern of any use in predicting development? So far, the answer is no.

BEHAVIOR-IN-CONTEXT

One possible way to get at the meaning of behavior is to observe behaviors in the situations in which they occur, yet here too we encounter problems. Consider facial behavior. Charles Darwin's initial observations have evolved into a measurement system that allows us to infer emotions from external manifestations in the neuromusculature of the face. Darwin and others, notably Carroll Izard and Paul Ekman, have argued that various behavioral movements of the face represent, in a one-to-one correspondence, the underlying essence or the emotional state of the individual.[8] I have called these manifestations *emotional expressions* and the essences *emotional states*.[9] An emotional expression is made up of a set of muscle movements located around the mouth, eyes, and eyebrow regions. Elaborate coding systems have been devised that allow, through the use of careful videotaping, measurement of facial expression. The relation between the different facial regions and the gestalt allows the coding system to specify which emotion (internal state) these different facial movements represent. Thus, if we smile when someone is telling a joke, the behaviors of the face may mean that our internal state is happiness.

Obviously, however, the set of expressions cannot possibly mirror, in any one-to-one fashion, the underlying emotional state. People are readily able to deceive others. Again, even the very young can deceive by masking an internal state through the manipulation of a set of external behaviors—and do it well! We mask our emotional expressions all the time.[10] In both children and adults the meaning of a behavior does not correspond to the underlying structures; the reality does not equal the essence. There may well be adaptive significance for the connection between facial expression and internal state being a loose one, especially when the social script requires competence in disengaging the essence from the reality. For example, parents tell their young children all the time that, although lying is bad, there are indeed occasions to do it. Mom says to the child, "Grandma is going to knit you a sweater for Christmas. I know you want a toy, but I want you to tell her that you like it even though you don't." It is quite clear that there are important social situations in which masking the face, dissembling the surface manifestations from the underlying state, is socially appropriate and serves to reduce pain and harm.

To complicate the issue, the context in which behaviors occur may not have the same rules for all people. Men and women cry for very different reasons. In my survey of what occasions elicited crying, men almost uniformly said that they cried most in situations that were sad. In a few cases men said they had cried at the birth of their child or in situations of awe. Women, on the other hand, reported that they cried when sad, happy, angry, and in awe. With such contextual differences, meaning between men and women, especially in this type of behavior, is likely to differ.[11]

Imagine a situation in which, while watching a beautiful sunset over the mountains, a man remains silent. The woman with him says to him, "What's wrong with you? Why don't you feel moved?" The man might be thought of as insensitive for not expressing emotional behavior even though he *was* moved by the scene. In other words, the meaning of his behavior was very different for her than for him.

So even though the meaning of a behavior is best studied in its context, if the context is different for different people, the meaning of the behavior may be different. In a study of children's play behavior I observed the relation between the type of toys boys played with when they were two years old and their school and peer adjustment at age six.[12] My interest in studying their play behavior was based on the observation that parents often are concerned if their young boys play with "sissy" toys, their fear presumably stemming from the belief that boys who play with "inappropriate" sex role toys are likely to become homosexual.[13] Given that children by two years of age show same-sex peer play, the concern that a young boy who prefers to play with dolls rather than footballs will find himself ostracized by his male peer group is not entirely without merit. So I classified toys by asking a group of undergraduates, as well as parents, to label the toys as male or female oriented. I found that some boys were more likely to play with girl toys than with boy toys; some were equally likely to play with girl and boy toys; a third group was more likely to play with boy toys than with girl toys.

When I first examined the data we had gathered, I found no relation between what toys the boys played with and subsequent adjustment. Children were equally likely to be well adjusted regardless of whether they played with girl toys or boy toys. But this was not the whole story. What would I find if I looked at the boys' behavior in the context of the environment in which that behavior was displayed? Next I looked at the data we had gathered about the mothers of those children; in particular, the mother's sex role identity. Some mothers had strong feminine orientation and preferred to view themselves in a feminine way while others considered themselves androgynous. The number of mothers who had a male orientation was too small to study in any detail. We now observed the boys' toy preference in terms of the mothers' sex role behavior. The findings were quite clear. The boys who showed female sex role toy behavior showed no social maladjustment if their mothers showed an androgynous sex role orientation but showed maladjusted behavior if their mothers had a traditional (feminine) sex role orientation. Likewise, boys who played with male sex role toys and who had mothers with a traditional orientation had no adjustment problem, but boys with mothers having an androgynous orientation did. Therefore, the child's behavior in and of itself had little meaning and was not related to later pathology. It was the child's behavior in its social context—in this case the mother's sex role values—that gave meaning to the behavior.

In some sense the essence, as opposed to the reality, of a child's behavior exists only as determined by others. Meaning is in the eye of the beholder. The child's behavior obtains normalcy or deviancy only by the context in which it is embedded. The idea that whether children show adaptive or maladaptive behavior depends on the nature of their environments has been called by Richard M. Lerner the goodness of fit model, and it indeed is a very powerful way of looking at how the environment provides meaning to behavior responses.[14]

THE CONTEXT OF OTHER BEHAVIORS

Most specific behaviors in and of themselves are of relatively little meaning. We use them only to reflect more basic constructs, such as crying to indicate sadness. It is very difficult to think of a construct that can be captured by a single behavior. For example, the constructs of attention, aggression, attachment, distress, and shame cannot be characterized by a single behavior and should not be measured in this fashion. What is required is an assessment of what behaviors cohere around the construct at a particular point in time and the nature of the organization of those behaviors. Following this, the set of behaviors characterizing the construct at one point in time might be compared to a set of behaviors characterizing the construct at a later point in time. Through this method of looking at the organization of behaviors, we may be better able to find continuity.* At the very least, however, the difficulty of this process illustrates the complexity of the contextual factors influencing both manifest behavior and the behavior's meaning.

In a study in our laboratory we looked at children's maintenance of contact with their mothers, or what we called the child's attachment toward the mother. What we were able to show was that the behaviors could be understood only in their context. Since the behaviors subsuming attachment as a construct change over age, one would expect to find little relation across like behaviors, a finding repeatedly reported. If, on the other hand, the construct is valid, one might expect to find different behaviors related across time, similar to what Emmerich found in looking at social development. Studying a group of children, we reported that children's seeking of close physical contact with their mothers at one year appeared irrelevant to close proximity seeking at two years. However, close proximity seeking at one year was related to non-proximity-seeking behaviors such as looking at their mothers at two years. If we assume that part of the attachment construct is related to the maintenance of contact, and if both socialization and growth pressures alter responses, then contact can be maintained either through close physical proximity or by visual regard. Thus we have a continuity in the absence of response specificity.

Observing sets of behaviors across different domains of functioning is another way of understanding what behavior means. For example, there

---

*Factor analysis, a statistical procedure, seems most useful in this regard. Sets of behaviors make up a factor or construct. Each behavior has a particular mathematical value that gives us an estimate of its relative importance in the factor under study. At different points in time factors may be highly correlated, but the behaviors making up the factors change or their relative importance changes. Thus, while there is no relation across time when one behavior is measured, the factor including this behavior may show consistency. An example of the use of the factor analytic technique for the study of early social development was first articulated by Walter Emmerich.[15]

have been many studies of infants' attentional ability. An infant is shown pictures, and how long the child looks at a picture is recorded. We also can measure the child's physiological response. One physiological response that has proven useful for infants, as well as children, adults, and even animals, is the change in heart rate. One of the most interesting findings is that when children attend, their heart rate slows down. The amount of attention appears related to how much the child's heart rate declines. So we have two measures of children's attentional behavior: how much they look at a picture and how much their heart rate decreases. Using these measures, we can study a six-month-old child to find out what the child likes to look at. Two pictures, one of the child's mother, the other a picture of a strange female, are shown to the child. The child looks equally long at both pictures, and since looking represents interest we conclude that the child is as interested in the picture of the strange female as in the picture of the child's mother. The behavior of looking does not seem to differentiate interest. We suspect, however, that the child may be more interested in the mother, and we have found that children show greater heart rate decreases when looking at a picture of their mothers than at one of a strange female. While the meaning of looking alone is insufficient to inform us about the underlying structure— the interest of the child—a combination of looking patterns and heart rate changes appears to do the trick. By looking at measures both behavioral and physiological, we may be better able to arrive at the meaning of a behavior than by looking at a single behavior alone. The problem of exactly what behaviors need observation in studying each construct, however, remains unsolved.

Unfortunately, measuring behavior even in context is problematic. It is clear that young children's behaviors are quite variable and that the meaning of the behaviors, at least as reflecting some underlying structure, may not be as clear as we would hope simply because we have not obtained a true measure of them. Such a problem might be readily solved simply by obtaining repeated measures of the child for the same set of variables, an expensive approach rarely approved by funding agencies.

Even if financial resources were to permit such research, this apparently straightforward task might be thwarted by the fact that children's behavioral consistency at the same point in time changes as a function of age. Young children's behavior is highly variable and becomes less so as they get older (although this too may be an artifact of measurement).[16]

There is considerable evidence that very young children's behavior is naturally variable; that is, their scores on almost any test are likely to change considerably from day to day. This may be due to the fact that young children are more influenced by environmental situations or immediately occurring events than are older children or adults. Thus the temperature or the size of the room, the color of the rug, or what they ate for breakfast may affect their "scores" more than these would affect an older person's.

The meaning of a response can be determined only after we establish whether that response is the true representation of the child's ability or capacity at that point in time. While we may not be interested in the behaviors themselves, but rather in the process or functions underlying them, we can deal only with observable behaviors, and these have to be reliable. Thus, to discuss the larger theoretical issues of development, it is essential that careful consideration be given to studies of reliability of the measures of the behaviors that we obtain. Unfortunately, this rarely has been undertaken.*

Similarly, since behaviors occur in particular situations, it is critical that those situations be kept constant to determine the stability of a behavior and/or its continuity. The measurement of a behavior or a set of behaviors in one situation at two points in time is essential. For example, maternal proximity seeking in a free play situation at one point in time may bear little relation to proximity seeking when the mother leaves the child alone at another point in time. Proximity seeking in a free play situation might be stable with proximity seeking at another point in time if the free play situation is maintained. Alternatively, a child assessed at home is likely to produce a very different score than in school because of such factors as anxiety or familiarity of setting. The strong form of situational determinism requires either stable situations or a full understanding of the context if we are to observe behavioral stability and continuity.

---

*Reliability has, for the most part, been an issue of the accuracy of the observer in obtaining or scoring data rather than the ability of the subject to produce the same response over repeated elicitations. When we think about this, it is quite surprising and upsetting that it is the case. It has been assumed that the response emitted by the child represents a true indication of the child's ability and therefore what is important is whether or not two observers would score the child in the same fashion. Thus, reliabilities always are between observers, called *interobserver reliability*, and rarely over the reliability of the child's behavior itself.

Consider the mother–child relationship. Since the nature of this relationship is reported to reside within the child as a trait or attribute, situational constraints only are useful to enable us to measure this phenomenon and its change over time. If, however, one allows for contextual influences, then the phenomenon and its changes may become more apparent. For example, in a study looking at the mother–child relationship in one-year-olds, we found that such external variables as time in the room, number of toys available to the child, room size, and familiarity of the setting influenced the infant's behavior toward her mother.[17] It may be the case that stability can be observed only when these contextual variables are replicated. This contextual model of development argues for individual stability or continuity only in the face of contextual stability or continuity. Thus an important principle of development might be that, given a consistent set of external events over time, some behavioral systems maintain their consistency whereas others do not. Unfortunately, little attention or care is given to these exogenous or contextual variables since our organismic theory emphasizes endogenous factors or traits as the cause of development. It is only a contextual model that acknowledges that behavior-in-context and the influence of context are as important as any measure of the child alone.

But even if contexts are the same from the observer's point of view, they may not be the same from the child's. Individuals create environments as well. Changing perceptions of the world will affect how the child responds to situations that may appear to an adult to be equivalent. Thus we need to discuss not only the context in which the child is observed but if and how we can determine the changes in the child's perception of the context.

We cannot assume that the situation defined by the adult is seen, perceived, or interpreted in the same way by the child at different points in development, which further confounds attempts to define continuity in change. American psychology has, for the most part, neglected the study of the context, concerning itself more with the questions of categorizing, observing, and assigning meaning to the organism's behavior; thus the emphasis in development on the organismic model.

The study of the context—or stimulus as scientists are apt to call it—of behavior is full of complications, the first of which is its all-inclusive nature. Anything can be a stimulus. Added to this difficulty is the problem of who shall define the stimulus. Barker[18] holds to the view that the stimulus can be defined by the experimenter in objective terms or measurable characteristics, for example, room size or color. An alternative approach is to define the situation in terms of the subject's perception of it. In either case, the task remains to specify dimensions used for differentiating stimulus situations. The situation can be defined in terms of physical properties that can vary along several dimensions, such as temperature or area. Situations also can be defined in terms of location, such as in rooms or buildings, or daily activities, such as washing and going to bed. The people involved in the situation can be another dimension. Classification across specific dimensions or combinations might even be possible. There is evidence to suggest that certain dimensions might be more interrelated than others; for example, people and emotions experienced appear to go together.[19] The enormity of the problem remains; the taxonomy of situations or contexts involves problems at both levels of characterization and interrelation.

In general, but more specifically in the case of infancy and early childhood, the context also may include other significant social objects—the mother, father, and so forth. Behavior measured in dyadic interactions, a type of situation, may be quite different from the same behavior measured alone. For example, smiling behavior as a consequence of a dyadic interaction may be quite different from smiling behavior produced when a child is alone, although the measurement of the smile took place in the same physical context—in her bed and in her room. Stimuli are not as they appear. We find, for example, that some of the things people see in the Rorschach test are the same but many differ. People presented with the same stimulus may see different things. What we perceive is as much a part of our development as is how we react or behave as a consequence of what we see. This is true not only as a result of individual differences but as a consequence of the developmental process itself. For example, many have shown that the scanning ability of infants varies as a function of age. Given a triangle, young infants are more likely to fixate on an angle than to scan the whole figure. Only after five weeks of age do infants fixate on all of the features. These developmental changes in what the infant fixates on when an entire stimulus is presented have important implications for the understanding of the meaning of the child's behavior toward it.

In the study of stability and continuity, individual as well as age changes in the perception of the stimulus or the nature of the context have consequences. There may be no stability in behavior from age to age because the context has changed affectively, even though the context itself is the same. Continuity may be unobservable not because the experimenter failed to hold constant the event in which the behavior was observed but because the event was perceived inconsistently by the child.

As we have seen, behaviors over time and different contexts can have little meaning.* This being so, I am forced to conclude that the error is not in the measurement but in the organismic model underlying our measurement strategy; the search for precursors or causes of later behavior may be a noble but impossible task. Since behavior meaning and organization lie at the heart of understanding the relation between earlier and later behavior, our empirical attempts to demonstrate it are less likely to succeed than I originally thought. While the idea of the continuous nature of development can be taken as a premise, it must, after fifty years of intensive study, remain just that, a world view. The question of the relation between essence and reality, posed over two thousand years ago by Plato, does not seem answerable by the study of development according to an organismic model. In its place we must find something else.

---

*While I have not discussed the problem of measurement for a contextual world view, I believe it is less of a problem. Behavior-in-context, the underlying metaphor of the contextualist, does not have to deal with the issue of change over time. As long as behavior-in-context refers to the unit itself, it does by definition have particular meaning. Hayne Reese put it this way when talking about the contextual approach to behavior meaning: "ask not what the behavior means at different ages, but what contexts the behavior occurs in at different ages."[20]

Chapter 7

NEWTON, EINSTEIN, PIAGET, AND THE SELF

———≈∘∘∘≈———

The above title is an analogy. Albert Einstein is to Isaac Newton as the self is to Jean Piaget. That is, just as Einstein's ideas about relativity overthrew Newton's absolutism, Piaget's view of abstract knowledge must give way to recognition of the role of the self in knowing.

I may, for example, know the sunset over the Chianti hills of Tuscany by having watched it, or I may know it by having read about it in a guidebook. Piaget's scheme implies that the latter is superior to the former. In Piaget's system of epistemology, when A becomes B, A is lost, a point already discussed in Chapter 3. Here A is practical or social knowledge, knowledge that requires the participation of the self, and B is abstract or formal knowledge, where the knower is separated from the known. B is a higher level than A. Yet modern examples culled from physics, our general model of science, show us that the self is indeed involved in knowing. Even in physics, where the role of the self was thought not to be necessary, Einstein and those who have followed have shown us that the self is necessary and inseparable from knowing.

The popular organismic model of development has not proved defensible, and a contextualist model must be considered. If we accept the relativity of physics, we must at least explore contextualism in development. The examples of physics, as I will suggest, seem to show again that there is no truth except that which is understood in its context. Extended to human beings, this idea indicates that knowledge exists not in an absolute form but only in its contextual form: what people know they know in context rather than in the abstract. Yet the organismic model as applied to knowledge tells us that ultimately the structures and forms of knowledge that develop are not necessarily limited or bounded by context. That, unfortunately, is a viewpoint based on ideas from eighteenth- and nineteenth-century physics.

If the self is involved in knowing to the extent that the model of twentieth-century physics suggests, then our knowledge, and hence much of our behavior, is determined much more by context such as cultural rules than by genetically programmed sequences leading to some unfounded idea of progress. As the self changes, so too will knowledge. Thus, what we know is both tied to and limited by what we are, what we hope to be, and what we imagine ourselves to have been.

PRACTICAL OR SOCIAL KNOWLEDGE

That practical or social knowledge exists can hardly be denied. There is no doubt that I can know of a Tuscan sunset through the overt experience of the self as well as by reading a book. Yet Newtonian physics—indeed the post-Bacon scientific method overall—would relegate practical knowledge to a status lower than abstract knowledge. For hundreds of years we have demonstrated a preference for abstract knowledge, usually thinking of it as the highest form of knowing. Knowledge that does involve the self has been considered suspect. Piaget, among many others, saw the acquisition of knowledge as beginning with practical knowledge and only later evolving into abstract knowledge. I believe that practical knowledge is a different form from, not a higher form than, abstract knowledge and that both forms are used by adults, depending on the tasks at hand.

Although a good characterization of the different types of knowledge and how we develop them still eludes us, our bias toward abstract knowledge is evident in many areas of thought. Not too long ago, I suggested to a young man deliberating about possible career choices that he consider the discipline of psychology. After some thought and further conversations, he said that he did not want to be a psychologist but would rather be a physicist because "anyone can be a psychologist, but not everyone can be a physicist." This statement seems to reflect perceived differences in the intellectual skills necessary to be successful in each career, and yet it is not clear that physics requires more intellectual ability than psychology. Nonetheless, the young man may have been quite right. Anyone can be a psychologist, because all human beings are psychologists. To live and interact with other people and objects necessitates knowledge of both oneself and the external world. Inasmuch as the study of psychology has the task of making explicit our implicit knowledge, the statement that "anyone can be a psychologist" is not altogether incorrect. However, a more accurate statement would be "we are all psychologists." As discussed by Kurt Lewin in the early 1930s, the relatively lower esteem of psychology may derive in part from the knower already having some knowledge about the known.[1] Thus, the degree of esteem accorded to a discipline may be determined by the extent to which what has to be discovered already is known. The history of science seems to support this claim: the various scientific disciplines have evolved in an inverse relationship to their proximity to day-to-day human activity, starting with the investigations of the heavens and moving slowly into this century's concern for the study of human behavior. The relation between knower and known affects how we value tasks; those that involve abstract knowledge are more prized than those that do not.

In Christianity, there are several texts that are not considered part of the core of the religion, such as the Greek *Gospel of Thomas* and the *Apocryphon* ("secret book") *of John*. Elaine Pagels,[2] in *The Gnostic Gospels*, describes the discovery in 1945 of a large set of texts reported to have been written around the same time as the four New Testament gospels accepted as the basis of Christianity. These texts had been banned soon after they were written, and those who believed in them were excommunicated from the Church and declared heretics. The Greek word *gnosis* usually is translated as "knowledge." The Greek language, however, distinguishes between abstract and social knowledge, that is, between "she knows historical facts" and "she knows me," or knowing through observation and knowing through experience. It is this latter form of knowing that is gnosis.

The *Gospel of Truth*, one of the discovered texts, describes how one group of early Christians, called Gnostics, believed that to know God required that they also know themselves. For the Gnostics, knowing was to be found in the process of knowing oneself; through the use of oneself, the barrier separating the knower from the known could be broken. This was heresy to the group now considered orthodox Christians, who "insisted that a chasm separates humanity from its creator; God is wholly other. . . . "[3] The orthodox view held that what was to be known, God, could be known only through some intermediary. The intermediaries were the true disciples, those to whom God had given authority. By breaking down the barrier between what was to be known and the knower, the Gnostics posed a threat to the structure of the Church and to clerical authority. Consequently, this form of gnosis was declared heretical and eliminated.

In thinking about the scientific enterprise or, for that matter, any intellectual enterprise, I cannot help being struck by something almost too obvious to mention. On virtually any topic, the views people subscribe to can be very different. Although disagreement between a learned and an ignorant person could be expected, disagreement between two learned people is surprising. These differences of opinion cannot be accounted for by claiming that one side is more intelligent than the other (although this might be the case); rather, such differences are more often explained by world view differences. In *The Cult of the Fact,*[4] Liam Hudson wanted to know where and how these different world views arise. How is it that two highly intelligent scientists, each possessing similar information, can arrive at discrepant conclusions? He sees that the answers to these questions may lie in the interaction between scientific and personal knowledge. In other words, we may need to ask what it is about individuals that facilitates their thinking about a problem in a particular way—to examine the characteristics of the knower so as to understand what is known. Certain characteristics of scientists may affect the truth value they assign to an event. In turn, how the scientist is viewed may influence the inclination of the scientific community to accept an event as fact. So the announcement of an unusual and unexpected discovery is more readily accepted when made by a well-known and respected scientist than by an unknown student. Pronouncements of eminent scholars often extend beyond their particular areas of expertise, yet they are taken seriously because of their prestige. The acceptance of what is known goes well beyond mere scientific and statistical probability levels; it involves the personal attributes of the scientist.

The scientist is intertwined with the science in other ways as well. As every sociology major is taught, one must be somewhat suspicious of an informant, especially when the informant is telling something that he or she wishes to be true. We recognize that our biases pose problems, so scientists try to show that they reap no personal gains from any discovery made. They know, for example, that we would be much less likely to believe a report that smoking is injurious to health from an investigator who does not smoke and believes smoking to be vile than from one who smokes. Ironically we are also more likely to believe a finding when it was predicted in advance (which surely means the scientist had a belief prior to the study) than when it was not. Predicted facts have a higher regard than nonpredicted ones.

The scientific enterprise usually assumes that the characteristics of the scientist are unrelated to the phenomenon investigated. A corollary to this is the belief that, when a relation exists between the knower and the known, the facts discovered are likely to be suspect. For example, if we were to give a personality inventory to two groups of scientists who held different theories and found that the groups differed along some personality dimension, both theories might be challenged. Consequently, one of the primary goals of Western science is to separate the scientist from the science or the knower from the known. Although relatively little research on the characteristics of scientists has been conducted, there appears to be a strong association.[5] We know, for example, that individual differences in aggression can be accounted for by genetic or socialization differences, with politically conservative scientists tending to believe the former and more liberal scientists the latter.

This diverse set of examples strongly suggests that although much of the scientific enterprise since the time of Francis Bacon has tried to separate, isolate, and distance the scientist from the phenomenon being studied, it may not be possible to make the knower entirely independent of the known. The knower is an active agent not only in one's social life but also in one's intellectual work. Such a view removes from the scientific enterprise the dress of objectivity. Rest assured, however, that such a position does not leave us adrift in relativism. What it does is lead us toward the realization that, indeed, "man is the measure of all things" (see below). To understand ourselves is to understand others, something similar to what some claim Freud tried to capture in his own analysis.

CLASSICAL PHYSICS
AND QUANTUM MECHANICS

The scientific method is designed to generate theory and predict events. These goals appear to be achieved in part through the separation of the scientist from the phenomenon being investigated. The experimenter's word and belief are replaced by a method. This distancing of the individual from the phenomenon of study through a commonly accepted method of empirical proof, reliability of measures, and logic represents a major event in the development of scientific method and practice.[*]

One founder of these ideas was Francis Bacon, who in the early seventeenth century offered the Western mind one of the first strongly empirical views of a philosophy of science. In *Advancement of Learning*, Bacon argued for more systematic experimentation and documentation: "They [the physicians] rely too much on mere haphazard, uncoordinated individual experience; let them experiment more widely, . . . and above all, let them construct an easily accessible and intelligible record of experiments and results."[6] In his first book, *Novum Organum*, Bacon challenged existing metaphysical views: "Man, as the minister and interpreter of nature, does and understands as much as his observations on the order of nature . . . permit him, and neither knows nor is capable of more." He argued that science must rid itself of the machinery established by Aristotle and must become as "little children, innocent of isms and abstractions, washed clear of prejudices and preconceptions."[7] In a word, Bacon counseled scientists to separate themselves from what they wished to study.

Toward this goal Bacon outlined his famous set of errors. The first is the *idols of the tribe*, which are fallacies considered natural to all human beings. Bacon rejected Protagoras's assertion that "man is the measure of all things" and tried to substitute a logical method free from the distortions of the human mind. This need for the scientist to become objective also implied that passions or emotions, anything hinting of subjectivity, needed to be removed: "In general let every student of nature take this as a rule that whatever his mind seizes and dwells upon with peculiar satisfaction, is to be held in suspicion; and that so much the more care is to be taken, in dealing with such questions, to keep the understanding even and clear."[8] *Idols of the cave* are errors caused by particular characteristics of the individual, stemming from prejudices, personality traits,

---

*On an individual level, intellectual abstraction serves to distance the individual from events or objects. One function of a symbol is to separate the thinker from what the symbol represents. This process of separation serves the same function for both the individual and the science. It is an attempt to know through the reification of the thing to be known and assumes, in a Platonic sense, that a reality or an ideal independent of the knower exists.

past history, or socialization. For Bacon such errors are a personal cave "which refracts and discolors the light of nature."[9] *Idols of the marketplace* are errors that arise between individuals as a result of differences in communication styles and language usage and imperfections caused by the commerce of ideas. Finally, there are *idols of the theater*, which are caused by the errors of others. These are the errors of dogma, the errors of "isms."

From this list of errors Bacon proceeded to explicate his scientific method of inquiry, with its hypothesis generation, empirical methodology, results, and conclusions. Bacon's view of science flourished, first in the founding of the Royal Society in England in 1660 and then in the work of Newton, whose views became the foundation for contemporary science. With the law of gravitation as its center and the use of related mathematical laws to explain the motion of planets, stars, and small particles, as well as the actions of people, Newton constructed a simple but bold synthesis of the physical world and the universe. The cornerstone of his entire system was the belief in the absolute nature of time and space:

> Absolute time and mathematical time of itself and from its own nature, flows equally, without relations to anything external, and by another name is called duration. . . .
>
> Space could be absolute space, in its own nature, without relation to anything external which remains always similar and immovable; or relative space which was some moveable dimension or measure of the absolute space.[10]

Newton's conception of the universe was as an absolute and orderly system, where space was like an empty room—basically fixed and eternally void—while time was like duration, always the same everywhere and at all times alike. This conception stood for more than two hundred years. Indeed, his view held so strong a sway over the minds of physicists that they could say: "In the beginning . . . God created Newton's laws of motion together with necessary masses and forces. This is all, everything beyond this follows the development of appropriate mathematical methods by means of deduction."[11]

Newton convinced us that, like some giant clock, the universe and its workings could be opened and looked into; and the opening and looking into, if done right, would not destroy the absolute orderly processes to be found inside. In this view a person could examine the workings of this orderly universe and extract general principles and laws that could further explain the observed relations. Newton's theories represent the most powerful example of the separation between the role of the knower and the known. Scientific objectivity, for Newton, rested on the belief that there is an external world "out there"—as opposed to an internal world, the I that is "in here"—and the task of the scientist is to study those phenomena of nature "out there."

The Newtonian universe, as it turns out, was imperfect. Toward the end of the nineteenth and the early part of the twentieth century, many scientists began to question its truths. The planet Mercury refused to conform to Newton's laws. Ernst Mach and Henri Poincaré, among others, challenged Newton's notions of absolute space and time. Finally, a radically new vision of the universe was provided by Einstein and twentieth-century quantum mechanics, accompanied by a totally new view of the nature of the scientific enterprise. Moreover, the new view of the universe and science brought with it a new view of the relation between the knower and the known.

In 1905 Einstein produced, in a single year, three papers that were to change forever the cherished Newtonian view of the universe. Suffice it to say that Einstein's revolutionary insight into the nature of relativity, together with Max Planck's and Niels Bohr's development of quantum mechanics, profoundly altered our understanding of the relation between knower and known, not only in physics but in chemistry, biology, evolutionary biology, and other scientific domains as well. No longer was the notion of absolutism to dominate our ideas of the universe. Instead the terms *relativity* and *probability* entered scientific discourse. For Einstein, relativity meant that the existing laws of nature were valid only when all observers moved at uniform rates relative to one another. Einstein described relativity in many forms, such as one in which he speaks of simultaneity as the perceived relation between two things: "So we see that we cannot attach any absolute significance to the concept of simultaneity, but that two events which, viewed from a system of coordinates, are simultaneous, can no longer be looked upon as simultaneous events when envisaged from a system which is in motion relative to that system."[12] Einstein came to understand that the nature of things was to be understood only in relation to the perceiver. That is, two perceivers standing in different places are likely to experience the "same event" as different.

Einstein's views of time, motion, energy, and space taught us that the properties of objects, time, and space were dependent, changing according to the particular system from which they were viewed. Events became dependent on probabilities rather than absolute certainties. The impact of these ideas on our notions of what was "absolute" and "real" was profound. Arthur Eddington, for example, suggested early in the twentieth century that the perspective of the knower to the known was not only of interest in analyzing the properties of objects but was essential to proper interpretation of any data on them: "When a rod is started from rest into uniform motion, nothing whatever happens to the rod. We say that it contracts; but length is not a property of the rod; it is a relation between the rod and the observer. Until the observer is specified, the length of the rod is quite indeterminate."[13]

Although this new view may have had little impact on the everyday lives of most people and their perceptions of the world of objects and people, the effect on the world of science was sweeping. No longer could one think of scientific investigators studying a phenomenon without considering their relation to that phenomenon. Phenomena no longer could be thought of as possessing absolute properties, as scientists once believed. Instead, the properties that they possess had to be understood as relative to the person who perceives them and to the agreement between the perceivers.

Modern physics soon went beyond even Einstein's conception. Max Born, Werner Heisenberg, and Niels Bohr, working within the discipline of quantum physics, conceptualized the universe in a way that leveled all remaining notions of an absolute and of certainty. For example, they concluded that statements such as that at a certain time a particle will be found in a certain place with a certain amount of energy or momentum were inaccurate and had to be changed to statements of probability. However, in the study of subatomic particles, quantum mechanics went even further, undermining the belief in a reality unaffected by human action. To some degree, the new physicists concluded, human observation and measurement actually created the phenomenon being studied. Quantum physics began to consider questions such as "Did a particle with momentum exist before we measured its momentum?" John Wheeler, one of this century's great physicists, asked one of the major questions of quantum mechanics:

> May the universe in some strange sense be "brought into being" by the participation of those who participate? . . . The vital act is the

act of participation. Participator is the incontrovertible new concept given by quantum mechanics. It strikes down the term "observer" of classical theory [Newtonian theory], the man who stands safely behind the thick glass wall and watches what goes on without taking part. It can't be done, quantum mechanics says.[14]

All in all, quantum mechanics had startling consequences. Not only was our view of the universe changed, but we could no longer describe the universe with physical models. The universe was no longer reflected in ordinary sensory perceptions; it no longer allowed for the description of things but only the probabilistic relation between things. Furthermore, the distinction between an "out there" and an "in here," or an objective reality independent of the observer, was not feasible because it was impossible to observe anything without distorting it. Finally, the new view of the universe destroyed our belief that we could measure absolute truth; rather, we could only correlate experience.

This new world view went beyond Einstein's personal belief system. Until the end of his life, Einstein resisted the notions of chance and probability and sought absolute principles and mathematical laws that could be used to predict events with certainty. His now famous statement "God does not play dice" reflected his displeasure with the new conception. Yet, as the nature of motion and the properties of matter, time, and space were all relative, epistemology, too, was changed. Referring to this changed view of science and knowing, Bohr writes that we have been

> taught that there exists an objective physical world, which unfolds itself according to immutable laws independent of us. We are watching this process like the audience watches a play in a theatre. . . . Quantum mechanics, however, interprets the experience gained in atomic physics in a different way. We may compare the observer of a physical phenomenon not unlike the audience of a theatrical performance, but with that of a football game where the act of watching, accompanied by applauding or hissing, has a marked influence on the speed and concentration of the players, and thus on what is watched. In fact, a better simile is life itself, where audience and actors are the same persons. It is the action of the experimentalist who designs the apparatus which determines the essential features of the observations. Hence, there is no objectively existing situation, as was supposed to exist in classical physics.[15]

Bohr's notion of "complementarity" directly affects the knower: the common denominator of all experiences is "I." Experience, then, does not mirror external reality but our interaction with it. The effect of such a conclusion on our role in knowing is profound:

> Transferring the properties that we usually ascribe to light to our interaction with light deprives light of an independent existence. Without us, or by implication, anything else to interact with, light does not exist. This remarkable conclusion is only half the story. The other half is that, in a similar manner, without light, or by implication, anything else to interact with, we do not exist! As Bohr himself put it, ". . . an independent reality in the ordinary physical sense can be ascribed neither to the phenomena nor to the agencies of observation."[16]

In a general way, we can see the self at work even within the scientific enterprise. Rather than the distant, disconnected world that many still believe characterizes science, the enterprise is filled with all the kinds of interactions between scientist and subject that we could imagine, including the theories proposed, the studies conducted, the data collected, and the analyses performed. Properties belong to the interaction of the phenomenon and the observer.

THE ROLE OF THE KNOWER

The role of the knower in mental activity must be acknowledged. Forms of knowing such as creativity, scientific discovery, and those great intuitive leaps that appear infrequently in each generation have been neglected in favor of the study of abstract knowledge. What is the role of the knower in such actions? The presence of large amounts of emotion, something that comes about only through personal involvement, in these actions should alert us to the possibility that the role of the knower may be critical in these forms of knowing. In a book entitled *The Eighth Day of Creation*, Horace Freeland Judson touches on this issue in talking about Linus Pauling and James Watson:

> To understand Pauling and Watson, you must remember that creativity is an ego drive, as much in science as anywhere else. I don't think there has ever been anybody doing great science whose ego

has not been involved very, very deeply. . . . Only Linus showed the willingness to take the inductive leap. Then, once he had the idea, he pushed it. The history of science shows that that, in itself, is perfectly justified—yet it's the same egocentricity that led him to collect thousands of signatures of scientists on a petition to ban atomic testings.[17]

Although Pauling dismissed this intuitive difference, another contemporary scientist said, "But didn't Linus also tell you that he has got more imagination than other people?" Whatever the processes, great creative leaps of thought, in science, art, or any other endeavor, may involve the role of the knower in some way not found in our everyday actions and thoughts. Rather than following Bacon's advice to avoid "whatever the mind seizes and dwells upon with particular satisfaction,"[18] the history of science and the biographies of people who have made significant contributions advocate the reverse strategy: to seize and dwell with passion on a problem and, perhaps, thereby find a solution. One can think of no better example than Einstein's remark when asked what he wished to do with the remainder of his life. He replied that he could think of nothing more satisfactory than to spend the next fifty years thinking about light!

So the characteristics of scientists apparently are related to the science they produce. One way to study this question further is to look at published work and see how it relates to the characteristics of the scientists who produced it. To do this, I looked at all of the articles published during one year in the two leading journals of child development. I coded each article on the gender of the person responsible for the study, whether gender was mentioned in the title, whether sex differences were hypothesized to exist, whether sex differences were analyzed, and whether significant sex differences were found in the data. Because the other features or characteristics of the scientists were not easily available, I chose the sex of the experimenter as the knower variable to use as the independent marker. As the investigation progressed, several facts emerged: To begin with, if sex differences were hypothesized, it was more likely that the sample would be divided evenly between male and female subjects. Yet the nature of our statistical procedures is such that evenly divided samples require differences in mean values of smaller magnitude to be considered significant. Thus, by hypothesizing a difference and selecting samples of similar size, the investigators increased the likelihood of finding the differences thought to exist.

I examined all studies reporting extreme sample selection—that is, having children mostly from one sex—as a function of the sex of the experimenter. There were seventeen extreme samples, twelve exclusively male and five exclusively female. When these were related to the sex of the experimenter, I found that male experimenters chose more exclusively male than female samples, but no difference existed for female experimenters. This finding may be nothing more than the result of an unusually small sample size. However, it does follow one of the more common socialization rules found for sex role behavior. In our culture, boys are pressured more into male stereotypes than girls are into female stereotypes. For example, females can dress in either a feminine or masculine fashion, but males can dress only in a masculine fashion. It is possible, then, that extreme sample selection for adult scientists followed the same socialization rules.

When I tabulated the number of studies where the sex difference hypothesis was confirmed, I found that male experimenters were correct at least three times more often than female experimenters. Several possibilities may explain these results. For example, male experimenters may be smarter or more analytic than female experimenters, but this is unlikely. Alternatively, male experimenters may be more likely than female experimenters to report a hypothesis only after the results are tabulated. Since hypothesis formulation supposedly should precede testing, female rather than male experimenters appear to be following the rules. Similar sex differences in rule-governing behavior have been found by others using different situations and more naive subjects.[19]

These types of findings alert us to the interaction between the characteristics of the scientist and the scientific facts that are discovered. Bohr's statement—"It is the action of the experimentalist who designs the apparatus which determines the essential features of the observation"[20]—takes on further import. Here, however, it is not only the action of the scientist but the personal characteristics, including belief systems, that affect the outcome of the experiment. This is not necessarily bad science, as a strict Newtonian might claim. It is simply an incontrovertible fact, one supported by modern physics. Rather than continuing to uphold the existence of an objective external reality independent of ourselves, it is time to consider a new model in which self and other in interaction become part of the unit of inquiry. Rather than ignoring such a relationship, it is better that we try to understand it through the specification of its nature.

Toward that end, we need to leave the realm of physics and see what happens if we study human beings using its new models. Does the self remain involved in cognition throughout our development as modern physics suggests? Or, as Piaget and other proponents of the organismic model would claim, does the self withdraw from knowing as we mature?

SOCIAL COGNITION
AND THE ROLE OF SELF

The epistemological issue of the relation between the knower and the known has been recognized by modern philosophers and psychologists for over fifty years.[21] For them, knowing involves the interaction of the knower with objects, events, or people. The structures of knowledge—that is, the schemes or models developed—are assumed to originate from this interaction. However, the mind of the knower, although formed through interactions, is believed to exist independently of the knower. Indeed, Piaget and others have thought that the degree to which the knower remains involved in the known is a measure of the immaturity or egocentrism of the knower.

Although it may be possible to separate the knower from the known for some forms of knowledge, in even the most abstract knowledge the known interacts with the knower. For instance, Gordon Bower demonstrated that whom one identifies with in a story will affect and change the person's interpretation of the story.[22] There also is evidence in memory research to indicate that memory is facilitated if what is to be remembered is made relevant to the self.[23] Language acquisition is another area in which the relation between self and knowing can be demonstrated. Although two-year-olds can demonstrate "on" or "under" knowledge by manipulating objects, they have far less difficulty when they use their own bodies rather than objects. Moreover, there is evidence to indicate that intentional verbs are applied to the self prior to being applied to others.[24]

These examples indicate that there is a difference in cognitive ability when the self is engaged, that there is indeed a form of knowing called *social cognition*, and that it serves us throughout our lives. The influence of the self on the outcome is no proof that a "factual" existence independent of the self does not exist, but it does point out that, in some forms of knowing, the self plays an important role. It is my view that cognition in general, that which we know and understand, represents a continuum of involvement of the knower with what is known. Social cognition represents knowledge where there is a marked relationship between the knower and the known. In other words, without the use of the self, some things are impossible to know.

But what exactly is social knowing? Social cognition has been defined in many different ways, for example, as social perception—the ability to disseminate different faces or to discriminate the face from a nonface stimulus. It has also been defined as the learning of social rules and obligations. In each of these cases the knowledge is considered social in that it applies to human beings, human attributes, and human products such as rules and obligations. Although this knowledge pertains to the features of human beings in some general sense, there is no reason to think that the knowledge formed should differ in any marked way from that explicated by Piaget and others for knowledge that is not social, because these features, perceptions, and rules require little or no knowledge about the self. They do not involve knowledge about the self, so they are not relative, and as such they can be studied like any other variable, for example, weight or volume. It is a Newtonian, rather than interactive or relative, dimension.

There should be no difference between studying social perception and studying other features of the environment such as weight, time, and duration. For example, children come to understand the notion of weight by interacting with objects, lifting them, and receiving proprioceptive feedback, and at the same time seeing them. Through development the child learns to conserve the concept of weight independently of transformations of the object and, in general, is no longer fooled by experimental manipulations of some of the object's properties. In the classical example of this type of study, a child is given two large balls of clay that are equal in weight. One of those balls is cut into five or so smaller balls, using up all the clay. The child is asked whether those five smaller balls will weigh the same as the one bigger ball. Up until a certain point of maturity the child will say that the five balls will weigh more than the single large ball. When a person thinks about the weight of objects, the self is not involved. The self can, however, be involved in the knowing. I can estimate the weight relative to my idea about heavy or light. When we think of weight in regard to another person, the other can be treated as an object: we can think about the features of another person independently of ourselves or in relation to ourselves.

Social knowledge also has been defined to include communicative competence, inferences about others, role taking, and emotional experiences such as empathy. Renato Tagiuri,[25] for example, has offered a classification of social knowledge that involves events inside the person, such as intentions, attitudes, perceptions, consciousness, and self-determination, and events between persons, such as friendship and love. These forms of knowledge are not independent of the knower or self because they pertain to knowledge that requires the use of the self. Role taking and empathy, for example, require that knowers put themselves in the place of another.

Social knowledge is thinking about interpersonal relationships. These thoughts involve the self in at least two ways. When I think about relationships, by definition they involve me; and when I think about relationships, one of the things that I may think about is what the other thinks of me. Recursive cognitions, or knowledge, can become quite complex, as, for example, when I think of what others think that I think of them. In his discussion of interpersonal relationships, Solomon E. Asch makes a similar point: "The paramount fact about human interactions is that they are happenings that are psychologically represented in each of the participants. In our relationship to an object, perceiving, thinking, and feeling take place on one side, whereas in relations between persons, these processes take place on both sides and are dependent upon one another."[26] Maurice Merleau-Ponty captures the spirit of social knowledge when he says, "If I am a consciousness turned toward things, I can meet in things the actions of another and find in them a meaning, because they are themes of possible activity for my own body."[27]

I have considered social knowledge as involving knowledge of others, knowledge of oneself, and knowledge of the relation between self and other. Knowledge about self and other are not separate processes but rather a part of the duality of knowledge. For example, Roy Bannister and Jay Agnew note, "The ways in which we elaborate our construing of self must be essentially those ways in which we elaborate our construing of others. For we have not a concept of self, but a bipolar construct of self–not self, or self–other."[28] The definition of social knowledge involves the relationship between the knower and the known, rather than characteristics of people as objects. By utilizing the self in knowing, we can differentiate when we are treating people as objects from when we are treating them as people. If the self is not involved, then the people are being treated as objects; when the self is involved, people are being treated as people.

An examination of cultural differences in these two types of knowing is beyond the scope of this book. But it should come as no surprise to find that cultural needs and values influence these differences. In fact, it may be a particular cultural mandate, such as a demand for abstraction and reification, that requires the knower to be separated from the known. Thus, as A. R. Luria and Lev Vygotsky suggest, different developmental levels or abilities are not controlled by some genetic program but chiefly by cultural requirements.[29]

That is, such abilities are governed by context. Evidence for this and for the fact that the introduction of the self into the acquisition or classification of knowledge affects the quality of that knowing is provided, at least in part, by an experiment by Nina S. Feldman,[30] who was interested in person perception or, more precisely, the formation of inferences by young children regarding the traits, motivations, and probable behavior of others. Earlier research had indicated that younger children tended to use what we call *featural knowledge*, descriptions of others' physical appearance or possessions, while older children described both physical appearance and the inner dimensions of the self, such as traits or stable dispositions. Such descriptions are recursive in nature and relational. In one study of five- and six-year-olds and nine- and ten-year-olds, Feldman showed that age was not necessarily the determining factor in the type of cognition used and the knowledge gained. The children observed on videotape four unknown peers who illustrated the traits of generosity, clinginess, physical coordination, and physical clumsiness. In one group the instructions the experimenter gave were made personally relevant by informing the young subjects that they would meet the children in the videotape after the study. In the other group this information was omitted. Feldman found that children who expected future interactions exhibited more and different inferences about the actors: "subjects appeared to be formulating a search in which a criterion of personal relevance mediated a change in proposition of statement types . . . used in descriptions of the actions."[31]

The relevance of these findings to the notion of involvement between the knower and what is known or constructed is clear. As the engagement of the self becomes more relevant to the task of knowing, social knowledge increases. Descriptions such as *nice, friendly,* and *helpful* are used more because they refer to the possible relationship the actor can have with the other. Feldman's study also provides support for the converse: that even with human stimuli the absence of the usage of the self results in a proportional decrease in the number of featural descriptions. In light of these findings it seems reasonable to believe that when the self is withdrawn from human stimuli the interactions with these stimuli appear little different from those not possessing human features. This intrinsically appeals to our notion that people can be referred to and treated as objects and that objects can be referred to and treated as people. The critical factor appears to be the degree of involvement of the self. Social knowledge and social action depend on the role of the knower. This is reflected in Fritz Heider's belief that "social perceptions in general can best be described as a process between the center of one person and the center of another person, from life space to life space. . . . A, through psychological processes in himself, perceives psychological processes in B."[32]

I would like to consider knowledge that does not involve the knower to be objective or abstract and liken it to Newtonian classical physics. Knowledge that relies on the knower is relative and, as such, can be likened to Einsteinian physics. Inasmuch as the study of the known excludes the knower in Piaget's genetic epistemology, it can be likened to a Newtonian study of objective properties. When the self enters into the known, the study of the knower becomes relative.

EMPATHY, EGOCENTRISM, PRIVATE ACTS, AND PUBLIC ACTION: A CASE STUDY

The class of knowledge involving private acts, including the thoughts and the feelings of others or acts involving relationships between people, must involve the self in the construction, maintenance, and form of the knowledge. Piaget and others interested in a more formal system of knowing would, of course, disagree. For Piaget, egocentric thought—thought using the self in an incorrect way—represents a lower, more primitive, less logical thought process. The young child, who assumes that his own perspective also matches that of the other, shows a lower form of knowing. Indeed, there are even lower forms, such as automatic or reflexive empathic behavior, seen in animals when one bird flies and all the rest fly or when one infant in the nursery cries and all the other infants cry. In a formal, abstract, logical, mathematical system what is called egocentric thought marks a less advanced, more primitive process.

The construct of egocentrism in Piaget's formal epistemology focuses on the knower's inability to separate personal feelings, thoughts, or perceptions from those of another. This is caused by an inability to understand that there is no logical necessity for what is felt, thought, or perceived by oneself to be felt, thought, or perceived by another. Although not stated, there is general support for the view that egocentrism, as an attribute of the organism, becomes less important with development and finally disappears as the adult knows that the other has feelings, thoughts, and perceptions different from one's own. However, to understand the role of the self, it is necessary to separate the process of using the self to know from the necessity for what the self feels, sees, or thinks to be the same as for the other person. I want to consider that in knowing, feeling, and thinking about others, we must utilize our own knowing, feeling, and thinking.

This form of knowing, what I call *empathy*, clearly marks the difference between ways of knowing, one focusing on current contextual adaptation and the other on formal, logical, and abstract reasoning. From a logical sense, as adults, we know that the perspective of the other, the feelings of the other, or what the other thinks does not have to be the same as what we would feel or think in that situation. While we adults can verbally state that logical knowledge, it is quite clear that we act in a very different fashion. In fact, it is very important for us to act as if there were a correspondence between our perspective and the perspective of another. Practical knowledge, rather than its more logical structure, operates contextually and therefore on the single case. It has as its goal both communication and exchange of information. Moreover, this exchange has to take place rapidly, giving rise to the assumption that the best guess is my perspective when interacting with another. This, of course, is what being social means. And it is, of course, the kind of knowledge that both has an immediacy to it and is related to the specific context in which it occurs. Empathy, as a case, can be viewed from its logical, mathematical, formal sense or from its practical sense, as in how people behave. Each view serves a very different model of development: Piaget's organismic structural approach versus the more contextual or pragmatic view, as expounded by Stephen Pepper and William James.

Empathy is the process by which the self is used to understand the world. This process emerges once the child develops consciousness, and we can see it by the end of the second year of life. Children and adults differ in the use of themselves as a source of information. Some adults rarely use it, and we meet them often. These are people who are likely to treat others as objects rather than people. We refer to people like this as pedantic, for when they speak to us they do not take into account anything that we may know. We say they are "speaking at us, not to us." On the other hand, we know of people who always are empathic. They remind us of people without selves, for they always are focused on the other. Such people often are overwhelmed by the pain of others. At this extreme such people cannot help others because they cannot distance themselves at all. How such individual differences occur is not well known. Heinz Kohut[33] suggests that parents can teach empathy by being responsive to and empathic about their children's needs. It is a likely source of individual differences. The evidence also suggests that women have more empathy than men.[34]

To understand human behavior, especially behavior that involves others, we need to understand the necessity for empathy, the ability to take the position of another, to utilize one's self to make statements about others: their beliefs, their habits, their feelings, what they have done in the past, and what they intend to do in the future. Empathy gives rise to feelings and thoughts. It is the glue by which people come to exchange information. When we engage in a conversation, for example, we utilize each other's knowledge systems and we behave so as to "tap into" that other system. Why should we be able to understand each other so readily, almost without effort, even when the speaker often does not know what she intends to say or how she will say it prior to doing it and the listener has to listen without necessarily knowing what the message will be; that is, the listener must listen and understand simultaneously? Such an information exchange system must rely on the ability of people to place themselves in the role of the other. In some sense, then, one major challenge in development is for the child to acquire a sense of herself as well as a sense of others' selves and the understanding that it is possible for these selves to communicate through the process of empathy. The child learns early to assume that another's internal life can be known by reflecting on her own. Empathy, then, is a practical kind of knowing. It is context bounded; the everyday mechanics of interpersonal life.

The loss of empathy, for individuals and for groups, always leads to pain. A child does not show empathy because he is brutalized by his parents. Empathy can be influenced by cultural values or current needs. Employing the self to understand another may be avoided when we assume, for some immediate need, that the other is "not like me." This always can be seen in the case of war when the other, say, a Moslem

Bosnian in the eyes of a Serbian neighbor, ceases to be "another like me" and becomes "the enemy." Group labels, such as Pagan, Gentile, Moslem, and Christian, are devices for separating self from other. On the other hand, there are cultures that are more likely than others to extend the idea of "like me" to other living creatures, such as birds or fish. The English were more likely to extend themselves toward their pets than toward the indigenous people of pretechnological cultures that they ruled. We Americans had established a society for the prevention of cruelty to animals long before we established rules about cruelty to children. These individual and cultural differences in empathy exist, and they point out to us the importance of this idea for our everyday lives.

The use of the self—whether it is called empathy or egocentrism—is not an immature thought process. It is a different way of knowing, no less important than the formal way of knowing.* It does not disappear and become replaced by formal thought. Even if I know logically that what I would feel if I were you does not necessitate that you feel that way, it is a good bet that it is how you feel, and in the absence of other information and in the need to act, such knowledge is useful and practical.

I am quite at ease in the belief that empathic thought is maintained even after the child learns that what is happening to the other may be understood by reference to the self but it does not have to be a correct understanding. Empathy, then, is not a failure or an immature process waiting for a new one to emerge. Gerald Gratch, in an interesting paper, directs us toward the difference between Piaget's representation of this formalism and the self-constructing knowledge system of George Herbert Mead. Gratch asserts that Mead attempted to understand how children's actions with persons resulted primarily in learning about themselves,

---

*From a developmental perspective, this form of egocentrism may not decrease with age. What may change is the child's belief that it necessarily follows that another feels X because I feel X; however, the use of self to feel the other's X does not change. Still the issue is not settled. It has been demonstrated repeatedly that given certain tasks very young children are not capable of assuming the perspective of another, whereas older children are, but the evidence does not indicate that the errors are egocentric. Rather, most of the children's mistakes are in considering what the other perspective is rather than in giving their own. If these results are valid, the developmental nature of egocentrism needs to be reexamined. A more probable explanation for the research results involves the child's ability to understand the task or the child's cognitive inability to find what the other's perspective might be rather than the child's belief that there is no other perspective but her own.

whereas Piaget "focused less on the organization of nature and social life and more on describing the growth of mental structures that are responsible for the particular ways in which children order their acts and the world around them at different periods of life."[35] In contrast to Piaget, for George Herbert Mead, the self remained an important part of the interaction. As Gratch points out, Mead's guiding metaphor was the "game," that is, the reality between me and you, whereas Piaget's metaphor was the "construction of reality." The central difference, then, pertains to the role of the self.

From the point of view of our model of development and the role of the self in that development, different forms of knowledge utilize in different degrees the self and self-knowledge. Similarly, Tulving's idea about different types of memories, those that use or do not need to use the self, clearly parallels the argument offered here—an argument for difference depending on context and predicated on current adaptation.[36] I may read about or experience a sunrise; they are different ways of knowing. The same can be said for knowing about pain. I can read about it and imagine it or experience it; they are not the same. It is not by accident that formal, structural, and logical systems of thought, as assumed by Piaget, for example, do not need a self who knows and see the self as interfering with knowing. It is part of an organismic theory of development, where old forms give way to new ones and the self in knowing gives way to knowledge without a self. Such a view is much like the Newtonian idea of what the universe was: a gigantic clock that runs on its own and can be examined undisturbed by selves. As Newton's view has given way to Einstein's, we need to turn our attention to the views of others who see the self not as a topic to be avoided but as part of the construction and communication of knowledge. This view of the self supports the contextual model of development as originally stated by William James.[37] We know in a context and for a purpose. This is the fabric of human experience, a fabric that may be distorted by methods of inquiry that require the absence of an active consciousness.

Chapter 8

CONSCIOUSNESS AND BEING

———————

I, for one, as a scientific man and a practical man alike,
deny utterly that science compels me to believe that my
conscience is an *ignis fatuus* [unreliable guide] or outcast. . . .
After the evidence of this evening, I will go away strength-
ened in the natural faith that your diligence and sorrows,
your loves and hates, your aspirations and efforts are real
combinants in life's arena, and not unimportant, paralytic
spectators of the game.
—*William James, "The Brain and the Mind" lecture,
Johns Hopkins University, 1878*

D espite how obvious it may seem that we are conscious beings, the
science of psychology continues to treat us as if we were not. From
a variety of sources, including "pop" psychology and empirical research
efforts, we are led to believe that we are bound by codependency, ravaged
by repressed memories, crippled by mistreatment as infants, limited by
genetics, destined to be molded by our genes and our environment.
Academic psychology and developmental models to this day do not take
kindly to the idea of consciousness, either as an active process that leads
to goals or plans in adults or as a guide for the child's course of development.[1]

Yet certainly since Immanuel Kant we have recognized the claim
that since "people have conceptions of what they want and should do in
order to reach the goals they have chosen, these conceptions, choices,
desires, and actions can be changed."[2] At least they can change their

lives. This is a fact that we see manifested in real life every day. It is possible for people to think about actions that will—in the future—have a negative effect on their lives and decide not to act in that way. I once knew a boy who stammered and decided to teach himself not to. He went away for the summer, and when he came back he did not stutter. When my friend who has marital difficulties decides to stop ruminating on what his mother did to him and instead opts to undergo psychotherapy to change his behavior with women, he is making a commitment to alter his behavior of the past to reach a new goal. Yet Phil Shaver, for one, who has argued for an organismic model, suggests that our choice of marriage partner is based not on a conscious decision but on our early attachment relationships.

No doubt, the history of psychology will show that the founding figures of the discipline chose to exclude consciousness intentionally, to avoid the appearance of being too philosophically inclined.[3] It is time, I believe, for the science of psychology to follow where philosophical beliefs and empirical example lead. Consciousness is central to understanding that the past does not have to determine the present or the future. The evidence that consciousness is an important aspect of the human psyche is ample enough to satisfy our scientific requirements.

The title of this chapter is intentionally drawn from Jean-Paul Sartre's famous book *Being and Nothingness: An Essay on Phenomenological Ontology*.[4] I consciously chose it, having remembered the work and having wanted to use it to represent my thoughts on the subject addressed in the following pages. Notice that I have used the words *intentionally, consciously, wanted,* and *my*. These words imply a belief in a self; more, a self who can think, remember, plan, desire, and execute action. Humans are active agents in their lives because they can think about themselves and their lives and, by thinking about them, change them.

We do not need to be servants of fate. Consciousness gives us the ability to think about ourselves, others, and our relation to them; to remember; to plan for the future; to change. Development over time cannot be orderly or dependent only on past events if we can think in the present about ourselves, our pasts, and our futures. Selves that are conscious must disrupt the connection between past and future.

"I am," "I want," "I will want," we exclaim, and our words give credence to the beliefs that we have memories of ourselves, that we are aware of ourselves, and that we have plans and hopes for what will be. We have a past, present, and future, and we can live in all three dimensions. I can remember what happened and correct it; I interpret what is happening now, and I can plan for a future, even one quite different from the past or present. Moreover, if we unite ourselves with some religious cause, we even can believe that we will have an everlasting future! Such truths seem obvious to me, but until recently cognitive science has virtually ignored the role of consciousness. Cognitive ability means more than a computerlike facility or an artificial intelligence kind of knowing; it must also include consciousness. Yet the organismic model is based on such a comparison. John R. Searle, the philosopher, has been an outspoken critic of cognition without consciousness for this very reason. Since René Descartes, he argues, we have rejected consciousness as an inappropriate topic for serious science. "I thought the major mistake we were making in cognitive science was to think that the mind is a computer program implemented in the hardware of the brain. I now believe the underlying mistake is much deeper. We have neglected the centrality of consciousness to the study of the mind."[5] We have also neglected its importance to the study of emotions and social relationships.

The psychology we have invented, especially that related to development, simply excludes consciousness. Most of our theories hold that the infant and child develop in a psychological space in which the self reflecting on itself, on others, and on the interaction between them is absent. Children are usually seen as passive to the forces around them, a view of the child that can be seen perhaps nowhere better than in psychoanalysis, another organismic model. Here it is believed that children's behavioral impulses direct their behavior and that the role of socialization is to modify and alter these impulses. It is in this struggle that the personality of the child is formed. The metaphor, therefore, is of struggle, conflict, and resolution; in particular, the socialization of the child's sexual impulses and Oedipal desires.[6]

But what if we gave to children the same active model of choice we often grant to adults? Children would be capable, with increasing degree, of thinking about their lives and changing them. If we give to young children the abilities associated with consciousness, we have, rather than passive organisms, active people in charge of their lives. Children thus do what people want not because they are forced to but because they want to. They are active participants in their own socialization. Rather than struggling with rules, they try to adapt to the rules. Parental rules and rewards and punishments become the material for understanding what the culture requires and a motive for action that arises from within the child's desire to be like others (and at other times to be different). Social control informs children that certain behaviors are appropriate while others are not and, at the same time, becomes the material they use to construct their world.

The Western Christian idea of being born in sin facilitates our view of infants and their behavior. Rather than inform them what it is we want them to do—that is, rather than enlisting their aid and support in their own socialization—we train children through rewards and punishment, a kind word or smile, an angry expression and physical hurt. Yet in everything they do, children express the will to adapt as we wish them to: "I wish to please my parents." "What is it I'm to do in this situation?" "How do these go together?" All of these expressions imply some active conscious agent. Having consciousness, they can change their minds, at times alter maladaptive behavior, continue behavior others think well of, and learn new ways of behaving. Active individuals like these can alter the past by remembering selective events and can produce a future for the most part independent of what came before. The conscious self can produce discontinuities between past and present.

Consciousness, then, gives us the hope that change is possible. The past may influence the present and the future but it does not determine them. Both children and adults are capable of change, not so much by focusing on the past but by thinking about the future. We plan for the future, we set goals, and we decide what we need to do to reach those goals. It would be foolish not to appreciate that early experiences have an influence on us, but it is also an error to assume that all our goals represent nothing more than predetermined desires.

Consciousness is, in fact, what makes us human. It is not thinking that sets us apart from most other animals as many believe but our ability to think about ourselves. Most animals are not self-conscious, and that distinction robs them of the volition and purpose that allow us to determine our own fate—and to alter it as we go along. It is consciousness that makes will what it is—a capacity through which we make choices rather than merely responding to biological impulses. With consciousness we have memories that help us make plans and control the future; we can produce the most radical of discontinuities.

If we want to understand how consciousness alters our fate, we need first to talk about how we think of ourselves. Like many important ideas, consciousness has been defined in different ways, so it is not surprising that it is difficult to find agreement on how it informs us about our models of change. I would like to argue that consciousness is one particular element in an integrated set of processes we call ourselves.

MYSELF AS CONSCIOUSNESS

As I sit here at the Hydro Majestic Hotel in the Blue Mountains outside of Sydney, Australia, sipping a glass of beer, the late afternoon sun shines and warms my skin. The taste of the beer is cold and sweet. At this moment I have no trouble thinking about myself. I know where I am and why I am here. I can tell the way I smell, and when I speak I can hear my voice; it sounds like me. The sun's warmth against my skin is comfortable to me. Sitting here, I can think about myself; I can wonder whether I will find a good restaurant tonight. I wonder about my appearance. Is my hair combed properly? As I get up to leave, I pass a mirror. There I see myself, the reflected surface of my being: "Yes, that is me," I say, fixing my wind-blown hair.

I know a great deal about me. One of the things I know is how I look; for example, there is a scar above my left eyebrow. I also know what I smell like, and my voice is familiar. Above all, I look familiar to myself, even though I have changed considerably with age. Pictures taken of me thirty years ago look like me, yet I know that when I look at myself in the mirror I will not look as I did then. My hair and beard are now white, not the brownish yellow they were thirty years ago. My face will be less smooth, and no matter how much I would like to see a very thin man in the mirror, I know now that when I look I will have to tuck in my belly to look like anything I wish to be. In spite of these physical changes, I have no difficulty in maintaining my identity—I know that is me! Identity can be maintained over large changes and transformations. Our own identity, by definition, supports our belief in our own continuity and, as such, supports our general commitment to see lives as continuous. It is one good reason to have consciousness. Consciousness is involved in all aspects of how we act. This is not to say, however, that what I know about myself is all that I am. In fact, consciousness is only one part of me; there are many other aspects that I do not know of. There are the activities of body: the joints moving, the blood surging, the action potentials of my muscle movements, as well as the calcium exchange along my axons. I may know of these activities as ideas but cannot find them in myself. For example, I have no knowledge of how my thoughts occur or why I feel one way or another, yet I am aware that I think and feel even without knowledge of how they come about.

I imagine myself as some giant biological machine capable of a complex set of processes—doing, feeling, thinking, planning, and learning. One aspect of this gigantic machine contains my consciousness. If I were an Eastern mystic, I might draw this idea as an eye, some seeing thing. Instead I prefer the metaphor of a protoplasmic mass, perhaps resembling the frontal lobes. For an excellent review of the biological bases of consciousness, see Donald T. Stuss, where both research and clinical evidence is presented to show that consciousness appears to be located in this region of the brain.[7] Consciousness is this mass that knows itself and knows it does not know all of itself. The me that recognizes me in the mirror is located in that particular mass. From an epistemological point of view, the idea that I know is not the same as the idea that I know I know. The consciousness aspect of the self that I refer to is that which knows it knows.[8]

Consciousness must be distinguished from everyday life functions. Much of our motor action, although initially planned, is carried out by the machinery of the body, which includes, by definition, self-regulation, organization, and coordination of various bodily functions. Although I know what I want to say (consciousness), the exact words I use, the sentences produced, their form, order, and style appear to be controlled by other mental processes, quite complex, that allow me not only to produce sentences but also to understand the sentences uttered by others. At times, for example, I say something funny but discover the joke at the same time as the listener. I am conscious of the joke, but not in producing it. This is not uncommon. Many times I have seen Woody Allen speak extemporaneously, laughing at a joke he made as if he had heard it at the same time as his audience. He has, I have noticed, a particular smile when he does so. If I ask someone to add a 7 to the sum of 7's that precede it (e.g., $7 + 7 = 14 + 7 = 21 + 7 = 28$, etc.), it is clear that the person carrying out this task cannot watch herself do the arithmetic. One aspect of the self, consciousness, has set up the problem or agreed to solve it; another aspect, what I call the machinery of self, solves it. Nevertheless, we need to lose consciousness as well. Those of us who play ball games or ski know that we can perform these complex motor actions only after we plan for them and *then stop thinking about them*; in a sense, by withdrawing consciousness from them. This is much like Csikszentmihalyi's idea of flow, which occurs when the skills we possess match the task requirement and we thus become totally engaged in the activity.[9] As I sit here and write, for example, I am totally involved in thinking about what I want to say. To focus my attention elsewhere, away from myself, I surrender consciousness. In the process I may lose my sense of time, forgetting to eat, only later discovering that I have skipped lunch.

The problems that we get into because of our consciousness is just one part of us and has been called by the Greeks *akrasia*, or failure of will. Last night, I promised myself that I would not have dessert with dinner, and yet I found myself eating a piece of peach pie and having a cup of coffee. Any explanation of this contradiction will need to include how the conscious me, which decided not to have dessert, interacts with the machinery of self to produce the outcome. Similarly, the elements of self clash perplexingly in our emotional life. Emotions include internally organized emotional states as well as emotional experiences. The experiences are part of our consciousness, but the state does not have to be—it is part of the machinery of self. I can be very angry at a friend for her insensitivity, for instance, and not be aware that I am in such a state. In an attempt to unravel the complex weave of the self into its individual threads, philosophers of the past have focused on, for example, the struggle between good and evil within the person—angels and the devil—as the definition of the self. Freud, for another, differentiated the self into the id, ego, and superego. More recent advances have pointed to the underlying brain processes involved in the conflict between our consciousness and the other aspects of our self.

A MAP OF THE SELF

Recent scientific research supports the picture of consciousness as one part of the self. The conscious element appears to have a physical location, although the exact site remains to be explored fully. Some have argued for the frontal and temporal lobes,[10] whereas others have been looking at the hippocampus and surrounding regions.[11] Self-recognition mechanisms apparently also exist in the great apes, such as chimpanzees, orangutans, and gorillas, but not in other animals, as far as we know.[12]

As an illustration, consider the description by Antonio R. Damasio, a noted neuroscientist, and his colleagues[13] of patients with bilateral damage to the amygdala, to the hippocampus, and to both. These patients were conditioned using a loud sound to produce startle and fear responses and having the sound associated with a visual monochrome image. The result of the study indicated that the patients with the bilateral damage to the amygdala could not be conditioned but had consciousness of the association of the light and sound pairing. The patient with bilateral damage to the hippocampus was able to be conditioned but was unaware (not conscious) of the association of the light and sound. The patient with damage to both amygdala and hippocampus could not be conditioned, nor did he have consciousness of the association.

Perhaps an even more impressive description comes from Karl H. Pribram, of a patient in whom the medial part of the temporal lobe, including the amygdala, has been bilaterally removed:

> These patients, just as their monkey counterparts, typically ate considerably more than normal and gained up to a hundred pounds in weight. At last I could ask the subject how it felt to be so hungry. But much to my surprise, the expected answer was not forthcoming. One patient, who had gained more than 100 pounds in the several years since surgery, was examined at lunchtime. "Was she hungry?" She answered, "No." "Would she like a piece of rare, juicy steak?" "No." "Would she like a piece of chocolate candy?" She answered, "um-hum," but when no candy was offered she did not pursue the matter. A few minutes later when the examination was completed, the doors to the common room were opened, and she saw the other patients already seated at a long table eating lunch. She rushed to the table, pushed the others aside, and began to stuff food into her mouth with both hands. She was immediately recalled to the examining room, and questions about food were repeated. The same negative answers were obtained again, even after they were pointedly contrasted with her recent behavior at the table.[14]

The brain lesion appears to have impaired this patient's ability to monitor her own internal state. Her consciousness or experience of her hunger was no longer available to her, although the state persisted. Of course it became impossible for her to regulate her state because she was never aware of it.

The clinical neurology literature has known for some time of a particular syndrome related to self-awareness. Such a syndrome includes loss of function and loss of knowledge about the loss of function. For example, Wernicke's aphasia results from a lesion in the left parietal temporal cortical region. A patient suffering from this syndrome not only has the loss of function but is unaware that he is unable to understand or to communicate with others. Babinski coined the term *anosognosia* to characterize this lack of self-knowledge and, more recently, Oliver Sacks, in his book *The Man Who Mistook His Wife for a Hat*,[15] has popularized this disorder.

In studying normal infants as they are learning language, I have run across a similar situation that seems to show how ability and awareness of ability can be separated. On several occasions an eighteen-month-old has come to the laboratory and, when talking, is likely to substitute an "F" sound for a "TR." This is particularly embarrassing for her mother when the child says "fuck" when she means to say "truck." The mother will often correct the child and say, "Jenny, truck." In such a situation, the child is likely to turn to the mother and say, "Yes, fuck." Being interested in this rather curious discrepancy between what the child hears and what she is saying, I have tried on several occasions to say to the child, "Oh, what a pretty fuck" rather than "pretty truck." On these occasions the child looks up at me puzzled and says, "No, it's not fuck; it's fuck." It is obvious that there is a discrepancy between what children hear others say and what they are producing or think they are producing. What they think and do is discrepant from what they think they are doing.

Lack of awareness of one's ability also can be seen in a phenomenon discovered by Weiskrantz, which he called "blindsight."[16] In this syndrome patients lack a visual cortex at least in one hemisphere. When a patient is asked if he can see an object placed in his visual blind spot, he reports that "I cannot see it"; that is, he does not have consciousness about the visual event. When, however, he is asked to reach for it, he shows that he has the ability to reach, at least some of the time, for the object. Thus, he can "see" the event but cannot experience his sight!

Michael Gazzaniga, in his book *The Social Brain*, has shown quite clearly the phenomenon that we can act and yet not know in a conscious way about the action. People suffering from severe epileptic seizures that travel from one cerebral hemisphere to the other can be relieved of part of their problem by cutting the corpus callosum, the bundle of nerve fibers connecting one hemisphere to the other. When such a patient is asked to reach under a cloth to feel with her fingers a number cut from wood, she is able to do so. If you ask her to raise her fingers under the cloth to indicate what the number is, she has no difficulty doing so. If, however, you ask her to *tell* you what number it is without looking at her fingers under the cloth, she is unable to inform you what it is.[17] In this study the patient examines the number with her left hand, which sends the information to the right hemisphere. Since speech is located in the left hemisphere, and since the hemispheres are disconnected, she cannot report what the number is verbally. Here is another example of how consciousness, at least as verbally reported, can be absent in spite of the fact that the subject knows, at some other level, the desired information.

So plenty of evidence exists that consciousness is one element of a self defined as an integrated set of processes. In the past scientists have viewed the self instead as a unity. This idea has led them to take signs of infants having a self as indications that they also have consciousness. Viewing consciousness as something that exists from the start of development makes it difficult to observe the separate consequences this capacity produces and thus its importance to development.

THE EMERGENCE OF CONSCIOUSNESS

Many scientists in the past have taken signs of infants' ability to do some complex tasks as indicating that they have consciousness from the beginning of life.* Although many abilities exist early—for example, the newborn must have some form of self-recognition, as seen in newborn or early imitation—the idea of me or consciousness is not developed until somewhere in the middle of the second year of life.

The fact that the frontal and temporal lobes of the brain evolve mostly through maturation over the first two years of life lends support to my belief that consciousness develops during those years (if in fact the lobes are where consciousness resides). However, the demonstration of consciousness requires, for the most part, language capacity. While con-

---

*There are earlier aspects of self, but the "knower who knows" is not one of them. For example, Kernberg, Stern, and Lacan all have claimed that young infants are conscious of their existence or the lack of their existence. But how can a child who lacks existence be conscious of anything? This is very similar to Otto Rank's notion of birth anxiety. Freud, in his critique of Rank, pointed out the difficulty of such views. For Freud anxiety was a signal and, as such, had to be experienced. Only the ego could experience it; "the id cannot be afraid as the ego can, it is not an organization and cannot estimate situations of danger." Thus there was no possibility of anxiety around birth or of consciousness of nonexistence![18]

sciousness does not exist at birth or even soon after, there are signs that it does exist prior to language. In an adult or older child, we could say, "Who are you?" or "Tell me something about yourself" or "Tell me something that you know that others don't know." Alternatively, following R. D. Laing,[19] we could see whether the child understands such statements as "I know you know that I know where you put your teddy bear." All of these questions assume consciousness.

Without language, however, children will have trouble explaining this idea to us. One alternative is to ask them to perform certain tasks that do not require language. If they understand the task given, it is possible to demonstrate that they have consciousness even though they do not have language. Thus, for example, in studying deception and in the research on theories of mind, we have been able to show that the child can intentionally deceive and to do so must place himself in the role of another. For example, Tom, a three-year-old, is shown a crayon box and asked what is in it. Tom says, "Crayons." The box is opened, and it contains candy M&M's. Tom then is asked, "What if some other child were shown the box? What would she think is in it?" If Tom answers, "Crayons," which he will, we know that he can entertain the idea about false beliefs. Such an idea implies that he knows that what he knows is not known by the other. Consciousness is implied. Unfortunately, even these studies require that children understand complex language, although they do not have to produce it. By focusing on minimum language production, we might be able to measure consciousness. Is acquisition of one's name proof of identity and therefore consciousness? After all, we are what we are called. The risk of accepting this as proof is that children may have been taught to use their name by associating it with a visual array (a photograph of themselves), without consciousness necessarily being present.[20]

Another language usage, a bit less suspect, is the use of personal pronouns, such as *me* or *mine*. Since parents do not use the label *me* or *mine* when referring to their children or teaching the children to recognize their picture, the use of these terms by the children is likely to be a reasonable referent of the possession of consciousness. This appears even more the case when we observe the children's use of these terms and how they behave when using them. I have seen a child saying "mine" as she pulls an object away from another child and pulls it toward herself. Since moving the object toward herself does not move the object as far away from the other as possible, the placement of the object next to where the body exists in space, together with the use of the term *me* or *mine*, could reveal consciousness. While useful, such a procedure still requires language, something a fifteen- or eighteen-month-old may not have at all.

A second area that appears to reflect consciousness, or at least a strong inner life, has to do with pretend play. Children around one and a half years of age, even before the acquisition of complex language, start to use pretend play. We see this when they feed their dolls or when they play at cooking on their toy stoves. These indicate the development of an inner self that acts, in effect, to say "I know that this isn't real, but it's fun to do anyway." This is action reflected on itself or consciousness.

Another procedure used to get at consciousness is to test self-recognition.[21] Following a procedure first described by Gordon G. Gallup, Jr., that used reaching for a spot on the face as a sign of visual self-recognition, my colleagues and I instituted a series of studies that observed the course of infant visual self-recognition. The data from a variety of sources indicate that infants, even as young as two months, when placed in front of mirrors will show interest and will respond to the mirror image. Children will smile, coo, and try to attract the attention of the child in the mirror. There is no reason to believe, however, that they believe that the image they see is themselves. Their response to images of other infants is no different from their response to their own. At older ages, when locomotion appears, infants on occasion have been observed going behind the mirror to see if they can find the child in the mirror. In addition, they often hit the mirror as if they are trying to touch the other.

Somewhere around age fifteen to eighteen months, it occurs to children that the image in the mirror, there, belongs to themselves, here. Consciousness is best captured by their use of self-referential behavior. As is well known, the touching of their noses, when they see in the mirror the rouge that has been placed there, seems to reveal that they know it is "me" there. Equivalent to uttering the phrase "That's me," it reflects consciousness.* What this consciousness will consist of, how we come to

---

*This ability to use the mirror to reference themselves often has been mistaken for children's understanding of the property of mirrors. There is ample evidence that when children are able to produce self-referential behavior through the use of the mirror-mark technique, they, at the same time, do not know many of the properties of reflected surfaces; for example, they cannot use the mirror to find an object reflected in its surface. What is important about the self-referential behaviors in the mirror is that they need not be a marker of general knowledge about reflected surfaces but a marker for the child's knowledge about herself.[22]

think about ourselves, and in what way or what descriptors we use will be elaborated and developed in relation to other emerging cognitive capacities as well as to cultural demands. Nevertheless, consciousness develops and can be readily seen in the child by the middle of the second year of life.

CONSCIOUSNESS, ACTION, AND FEELING

With the emergence of consciousness in the second year of life, we see vast changes in both children's emotional life and the nature of their social relationships. With consciousness children can act empathically and thereby alter their social behavior in accordance with the needs and desires of others; they are truly social. With consciousness the child can feel what I have called self-conscious emotions, like pride at a job well done or shame over a failure.[23] Consciousness allows children to be able to determine the course of their lives. It provides the mechanism for altering the past though the reconstruction of history. Perhaps more important in terms of the perspective that earlier events cause later ones, consciousness forces us to review the world of socialization, as articulated by Freud and the psychoanalysts, which sees children in a struggle with their caregivers, a model that fails to appreciate children as active organisms capable of producing and therefore changing their own socialization. Such a passive model fits well into the view of development as a fixed and determined unfolding where earlier events influence later ones. If, however, we reject this model of socialization, we also reject the implicit overall model of development it supports. Once people have consciousness; once they can ask about themselves; once they can think of themselves in the past, in the present, and in the future; once they have the capacity to make plans, they are capable of reconstructing their life, even altering past events as they affect the present. This process is likely to be an ongoing one across the entire developmental time frame. When the three-year-old feels pride in a deed accomplished, that feeling is likely to motivate the child to form plans to achieve more of it, to give up behaviors that do *not* elicit the feeling, and to seek out behaviors that do. In like fashion, those behaviors that cause shame are likely to be altered or eliminated. Consciousness leads to cognitive–emotional structures and feelings that people can use to alter the course of their lives.

How individuals are likely to interpret the moral value of what they do or think depends on many factors. In my book on shame,[24] I show how all the evaluative emotions have to do with consciousness. First, consciousness related to some goal, standard, or rule is necessary for these emotions to occur. Second, consciousness is necessary for us to have knowledge of our performance and to compare our performance to our standards. Third, consciousness is necessary for us to feel responsible for the success or failure of our action toward a standard. I may be happy that I have won a lottery, but I am not proud of having done so because winning did not come about through any action on my part. Thus, to be proud we have to think about whether our action caused the achievement of the goal. Finally, consciousness is involved in our evaluation of ourselves relative to success or failure. Failing and thinking that we are in general no good gives rise to the emotion of shame. On the other hand, thinking about the specific actions leading to the failure gives rise to the emotions of guilt or regret. In all of these emotions the need for conscious processes, as well as meta-representations that also involve consciousness, is present.

What is important in this process is that through consciousness children are able to develop emotions that affect their own behavior. Thus when children feel proud of what they do, they are provided with an internal motive to do more of the behavior or activity that leads to that feeling. Feeling guilty or shameful acts in a similar fashion. In other words, the reinforcing control of the environment is transferred from parent to child. Children can control their fate, alter their behavior, and undo past events by utilizing these emotions, emotions that derive from their own consciousness. In fact, I would go so far as to say that only conscious creatures can feel pride and shame, and because most other animals do not possess consciousness, they do not possess these emotions. My cat and dog do not feel shame when they do something they have learned brings punishment. What they have, if anything, is the fear associated with the action and punishment. The same is true for the human child prior to three years of age.

The relation between conscious emotions and social behavior can be seen in the ability to lie. In some recent studies we asked children not to look at a toy and then provided them the opportunity to do so when we were not watching them. Most children looked at the toy, but when questioned as to whether or not they did so, the vast majority of them lied. Sixty-five to seventy percent of two-and-a-half-year-old children lied when asked. Not only were the children capable of lying in response to the experimenter's question, but they were able to mask their facial and body postures so that it was difficult to tell without careful observation that they were lying. To deceive, the child first had to know and remember that she was asked not to look; the child had a memory of what she was asked about. Moreover, the child had to know that telling the truth would get her into trouble, indicating that the child had knowledge of what her behavior would cause. Finally, these young children had to know that they knew something that the experimenter did not know and would not know if they did not tell them. This set of knowledge suggests an active consciousness engaged in the intention to deceive. While other interpretations are possible, it is quite clear that consciousness plays an important role in the child's behavior. Consciousness also brings identity. If I am conscious of myself, I must be conscious of the self of others. Consciousness affects our understanding of a person and the personage of others. It is therefore basic to mature human relationships.

My view of mature human relationships requires consciousness. As George Herbert Mead and Harry Stack Sullivan[25] were well aware, relationships are possible only through the negotiation of two or more conscious selves. Interactions between conscious organisms lead to a relationship through awareness of each self, each other's self, and the space occupied by both selves. What we mean when we refer to mature human relationships is the level that includes what organisms think about themselves and the other, the desire to share, the use of empathy to regulate the relationship, and the ability to anticipate the needs of the other. As Robert A. Hinde[26] has indicated, true human relationships require those mental processes that allow two people to think of the other as well as themselves. Consciousness also involves ego boundaries. When we consider ego boundaries, we need to make reference to the child's growing understanding of privacy, as well as the child's need to become a "we"; that is, to join in a relationship with others.[27] Without this skill, this capacity of consciousness, we may talk about relationships but we certainly cannot be making reference to mature adult ones. Animal relationships do not need this skill, and neither may relationships in infancy that occur prior to the acquisition of consciousness. The meaning of the term relationship, therefore, is not the same from organism to organism or at different points in a child's development. Human relationships are likely to exist in a rather limited form between adults and children prior to the child's development of consciousness. Uniquely mature human relationships arise from interactions only after the development of consciousness in the child.

We must be careful, then, when we talk about the mother–infant relationship, to understand that this is a different type of relationship from the mother–child relationship. From this point of view the achievement of an adult human relationship has a developmental progression. By two years of age most children have consciousness and their relationships now approximate more closely those of adults. Margaret S. Mahler's concept of individuation is relevant here, for—as she has pointed out—only when the child is able to become an individual, to stand alone, can it be said that the child can form a more mature relationship.

Such an analysis raises the question of the nature of the child's relationship prior to consciousness. For me a preconsciousness relationship is a complex social species-patterned process, which is imposed by the caregivers and which, through adaptive processes, may exist in the human infant. This imposed or socialized complex patterned system ultimately gives way to a mature relationship in which the child joins in the socialization process through the advent of consciousness.

Attachment theorists have given some thought to this problem. In particular, Mary S. Main and her colleagues, as well as Inge Bretherton, have returned to a more cognitive view of attachment, as suggested originally by John Bowlby. They utilized his schema, called a *working model*, as the basis of an attachment relationship. By focusing attention on the child's cognitive construction, rather than just on the interactive pattern of the mother and child, the theory of attachment involves consciousness. For example, Bowlby states, "The model of the attachment figure, and the model of the self, are likely to develop so as to be complementary and usually non-conforming. Thus, an unwanted child is likely not only to feel unwanted by his parents, but to believe that he is essentially unwanted."[28] If this is so, then attachment as a cognitive process does not emerge until the middle of the second year of life.

Relationships are based on consciousness, which gives rise to the ability to consider not only yourself but others and the relationship of you to them and them to you. When I say that "I know that you know that I know you did not read the newspaper today," I am capable of forming a relationship because I think I have knowledge of the two selves that form the relationship. My social life is dependent, therefore, on consciousness. In the same way, my knowledge of your knowledge of me provides me with the opportunity to change what you believe about me. Social interaction can be enhanced or altered through this action. In the case of animals, where relationships are dependent only on old action patterns, the opportunity to alter one's current relationships, freeing them from the oppression of the past, is limited.

This analysis suggests that consciousness gives rise to internalized emotional behavior, identity, and the ability to form and maintain relationships. These abilities define an active organism, one capable of remembering her past and modifying it to serve the present or future, of constructing goals and plans for the future, and of going into therapy so as to change. Consciousness gives rise to goals, and goals allow us to change.

Recent interest in the idea of a conscious self makes it clear in hindsight that excluding consciousness from the psychological study of the self was a foolish digression. I take as a credo, then, the belief that we are not some unconscious creatures, controlled solely by biological forces within or environmental forces without. We are not destined to live out our lives uninformed, without intentions or desires, and unaware of ourselves. Lives are influenced by many forces: by their evolutionary–biological history, by the reinforcing properties of others, and, perhaps most important, by consciousness.

Chapter 9

ADAPTATION AND THE NATURE OF SOCIAL LIFE

———⟨∘⚬∘⟩———

Most of us grew up believing that our earliest relationships seal our fate by determining who we will be when grown. Our mothers, in particular, are held to be the most critical figure for determining our social relationships. It is no wonder that my friend (in Chapter 3), having difficulty in his marriage, would say, "I wonder what my mother did to me." Such a view is emblematic of the way we view the role of our mothers in our lives. Such a view of mothers is suggested by Sigmund Freud's work with humans and Harry F. Harlow's work with monkeys. We take the mother's impact as an accepted fact. But such a view of motherhood has recently come under review as our concept of family has been altered and as the data on her role in a child's life has failed to support her presumed singular importance. It is time to reexamine the idea.

I find it strange that the myth of attachment theory, one of the best examples of an organismic model, lingers on among many people like my unhappy friend and, unfortunately, among social policy makers. This is due in part to our belief that individuals have traits and that these traits are derived from earlier experiences, in particular those with our mothers. Because of these beliefs, much research has been directed at mothers, and at first glance the findings appear to support attachment theory. I believe, however, that much of that evidence can be refuted, that research along other lines of inquiry would show the merits of a theory based on social context and current adaptation. To uncover the limitations of attachment theory and see how social adaptation rather than traits affects our social lives, we must scrutinize attachment theory in some detail.

Perhaps nowhere else is the organismic model of development used more than in explaining human social development. Attachment theory, as articulated by John Bowlby and Mary Ainsworth, epitomizes this traditional model of development: the early mother–child relationship produces a certain type of child who has a certain characteristic; one child is secure, while another is insecure. This early experience creates in the child a kind of trait or characterization, which in turn determines the child's subsequent relationships, including those with fathers, siblings, and peers.[1]

In attachment theory we can see almost all the features found in the organismic model of development, so dislodging attachment theory also helps us challenge the foundation of the organismic model of development. For example, that earlier events affect later ones is seen in the belief that what happens in the early months of life affects the child's attachment relationships at one year and that the one-year trait affects what happens to the child later—even extending into adult romantic and parenting life. There is progress and order, with the child–mother interaction leading to secure attachment and some characteristic, such as ego strength or mental health, and then this trait leading in turn to healthy peer and adult relationships.

Such a theory of social and emotional development has captured the attention of Western society since, in its general form, it resembles object relations psychoanalytic theory, a theory of development extending in one way or another back to the founding of the psychoanalytic movement at the beginning of the twentieth century. This theory both supports the traditional model of development, what I have called the organismic model, and informs us how powerful such ideas about how development works are for us all.

For many reasons, as we have already seen, I favor a theory of contextual adaptation rather than a trait theory. In the social realm the most important reason is that by nature humans are social animals. From the moment of birth the child is surrounded by other conspecifics, a small number of whom share the child's gene pool, a larger number of whom will influence the child and in turn be influenced by her, and, finally, the largest number of whom form the background in which these other interactions will take place. The smallest group we call the family. The larger comprises lovers, friends, acquaintances, and even strangers. The largest group is the culture itself. It is within this total array that the developmental processes occur. Given that the major task of the newborn is to adapt to this environment of people, it seems reasonable to assign to humans the feature of sociability. Because newborns must live in this social world, much of their sensory and cognitive abilities center around making sense of a variety of people. To this adaptation the newborn brings many skills and biological structures.[2]

A social network is an interconnection of events and people, and it is to this network that we look to observe the environment to which the infant adapts. This network includes significant others beyond family: friends, teachers, and eventually mates. We can think of this array as a set of interconnected networks. The family is the nuclear one and is embedded in other networks that form larger reference groups, such as religious groups, countries, or cultures. These networks exert influence on each other. They form what Urie Bronfenbrenner has called the "ecology of human development."[3] Moreover, it is reasonable to assume that each of these separate networks, as well as the entire system of networks, operates as a complete system. So to understand this ecology, we need to know something about systems theory, how large numbers of elements are related to each other, a subject broached later in this chapter. First, let us examine the more widely accepted theory, which ignores social systems in favor of a single relationship and trait.

THE ATTACHMENT THEORY
OF DEVELOPMENT

Attachment is the only type of relationship that has been studied in any detail in early childhood. Attachment is an affective bond that provides the child with a secure base that allows the child to explore the world and to develop adaptive social and emotional skills. The concept of attachment allows for only two types of general relationships, attached and not attached; within attached there are secure and insecure types.[*]

That the mother, through her unique biology, held a special role vis-à-vis her child surely was obvious for ages, but exactly when theories about the importance of the mother were first developed is difficult to

---

[*]Recently a disorganized type has been identified, but I suggest it is much like not attached. Within attached there are three types—secure (called type B), avoidant (called type A), and ambivalent (called type C). Most studies compare B versus A and C groups.

state. Certainly by the turn of the century psychoanalytic theory had described the central role of the mother in the child's life. Indeed attachment theory is an extension of that view as first expounded by Freud. Freud's particular organismic model specifies that the mother is the first and primary factor in the child's social life and that all subsequent relationships are affected by it: if the mother–child relationship is a good one, the child will have a good social development; conversely, if the mother–child relationship is poor, the child will have poor social relationships.

Fixed Sequence

Attachment theory supposes a fixed sequence, as does the organismic model of development: the infant first forms a relationship with the mother; from this the child acquires a characteristic; and from this all subsequent relationships follow. These include relationships with the father, siblings, peers, and even grandparents. While the initial attachment relationship with the mother is argued to be the primary one, the child's attachment relationships with others has not been tested. There probably are thousands of studies in the literature about the child's relationship with the mother, but to date only seventeen known studies have compared the child's attachment to the father. Nor do we have much information on the child's attachment to other people, including siblings and grandparents, although there is clear evidence that they do form attachments with them. Attachments are possible toward child-care workers in daycare settings,[4] and several studies indicate that children can form an attachment relationship to objects, such as their security blanket or favorite toy, and that these attachment relationships can be used by the child as a base for comfort when distressed.[5] Children can be attached to more than one person at a time, and there are data to show that a child can have an insecure attachment to the mother but a secure one to another person.[6] The fixed sequence idea cannot be demonstrated.

The fact that multiple attachments have not been studied must be a function of cultural bias. Studies of other cultures concerning the important role older siblings, uncles, aunts, and grandparents play should alert us to the fact that, at least for some cultures, these people also should be included in a list of possible attachment objects.[7] It would seem, then, that the number and nature of attachment figures are dependent on the structure of the culture. In cultures where the older female sibling is in charge of the infant, there is little question that the child forms an attachment to her as well. While infants cannot survive without at least one figure caring for them, the nature and number of others involved in the child's life seem to be a function of the values of the larger social system.

Determinism

The theories of Freud and Bowlby assume that later social experiences are determined by earlier ones, particularly the relationship between mother and child. This view still holds sway, manifested in the belief that the mother–infant attachment determines the child's later peer relationships as well as later romantic ones.[8] While much has been made of the deterministic nature of early relationships, the data are rather limited and various alternative explanations remain unexplored. Such a deterministic view of early mother–child relationships is best exemplified by Harry Harlow's studies of motherless monkeys who were at risk for dysfunctional peer relationships as well as for later mothering problems.[9] While the determinism seen in the Harlows' data did lend support to a theory of attachment relationships, more recently it has been pointed out that the deleterious effect reported by Harlow was not caused by the lack of mother–infant relationships but rather by the complete social isolation in which the monkeys were raised. Baby monkeys raised with other babies showed few of the effects originally reported.

There is little reason to believe that the infant cannot form multiple attachments at the same time. In cultures that allow for multiple attachments, they occur. In cultures that leave the child alone with the mother, we are apt to see a more sequential adjustment. Even more important, repeatedly research has shown that peer development, rather than being determined by the mother–child relationship, evolves in a parallel way, giving rise to at least a dual affect system.[10] Thus when exposure to peers is culturally sanctioned I view peer relationships as developing in tandem with the mother–child attachment, not as being determined by it. With the growth of infant day care we are witnessing a mass social structure change, and its implications for our theories and social practices are becoming increasingly apparent. Recent battles over the effects of day care reflect the struggle now occurring between our developmental theories and social policy. Although there is a bit of equivocal evidence to support the deterministic effect of one relationship on another, the majority of evidence does not support this idea. This is not to say that one relationship cannot exert an effect on another. Indeed, such an effect is envisioned. The difference between the position as proposed by the attachment theory and a systems theory approach is the deterministic nature of the effect. Stephanie Schaeffer and I[11] have argued for alternative explanations of why an insecure relationship with the mother is associated with poor peer relationships. In effect, poor mothering includes preventing the child from having successful peer relationships. It is not a direct cause of them, seen especially when children are given peer experience independent from their mothers.

Traits

The controversy surrounding the nature of traits or enduring aspects of personality that has dominated much of contemporary thinking on the topic of personality comes up again in considering the effect of one relationship on another. For me this area accounts for the major difference between the organismic and contextual models.

Attachment theory proposes that the mother–infant relationship endows the infant with a trait or characteristic that determines subsequent relationships. While the nature of this trait has not been clarified, it has been associated with ego skills.[12] Whatever its nature, it is the presence or absence of this trait within the child that influences other relationships. Embedded in this trait concept is the idea that there are critical periods in a child's life. In attachment theory the mother–infant relationship in the opening months of life is assumed to be critical; if this relationship is inadequate, then all subsequent relationships will be affected. However, although it is seldom recognized, the relationship between mother and child does not always remain the same during the critical early months—and when it changes it does so especially in response to environmental stress. It is difficult to see how a definable trait can be created by an indeterminate relationship.[13]

The trait idea also provides a mechanism for the deterministic nature of this theory: one relationship creates a trait in the child that is not easily affected by experience, and the child then brings this trait to bear on the child's next relationship. Certainly from an experiential point of view early relationships appear to exhibit a strong influence on later ones, and a personality trait seems to be a reasonable mechanism for linking these experiences. However, we now have sufficient data to show that this theory simply does not hold up. Again the motherless monkey provides important information. The poor mothering behavior of motherless monkeys was used as an example of the consequence of a poor mother–child relationship. But, as pointed out by others, including Harry Harlow himself, after their first children these motherless monkeys were quite normal in their mothering. The more time a mother spends with the first child, even though she maltreats it, the better mother she appears to be with the second. A similar finding comes from the peer relationships of abused infants. If maltreated or abused infants have poor attachment relationships with their mothers and this leads to a deficiency in a trait, according to attachment theory they should end up having poor peer relationships. They do not. When given positive experiences with peers, they thrive.

When there are no intervening positive peer experiences, a poor relationship with the mother may be related to poor peer relationships only in that such mothers may prevent the infant from having good peer experiences. Given that the mother in our culture facilitates early peer contact, her failure to do so will result in the absence of contact and, as a consequence, the development of inadequate peer interaction skills. In this case poor attachment and poor peer relationships are related, but one does not cause the other in a traitlike way. Rather, it is how the mother helps construct the social context of her child that is at work. Attachment relationships seem to exert their influence more in the construction of environment; attachment classification of a child remains stable only as long as the environment in which the child functions remains stable.[14]

The fact that attachment changes when the child's environment changes casts doubt on whether a trait is created at all. If attachment changes, then the trait it creates should change as well, yet a trait is defined as an enduring feature that, once it is created, does not change easily and does not depend on the environment. So it is logical to conclude that what changes when attachment changes is not a trait within the child but simply the child's behavior as driven, at least in part, by the nature of the environment. The attachment classification of the child—whether the child behaves in a secure or insecure way—can be seen as a manifestation of the environment rather than of the child. A child's competence later in life may reflect not a secure early attachment but a positive environment at that later point in life. The relation between the child's earlier and later behavior may not be mediated by the attributes of the child but by the environment at both earlier and later times. If the environment remains bad, the child remains bad; if the environment remains good, the child remains good. If the environment changes from good to bad, then the child changes from good to bad. Unlike a trait attribute located in the child, the behavior of the child reflects the context in which it occurs.

Certainly many individuals—and consequently society as a whole—would become open to an alternate theory of development if they realized how questionable are the scientific truths on which attachment theory depends. The six findings I examine on the following pages should alert us to the problems linking the early mother–child relationship to all subsequent development and reveal that alternate views must be considered. In the study of social development the belief that children's earliest social experiences impact on their later life and that these early social experiences, for the most part, are caused by parenting styles, in particular the mother's, are spoken of as proven facts. In actuality there is considerable reason to doubt the validity of each of them.

FALLACY AND FAITH

The Face as an Innate Releasing Mechanism

It is commonly believed that the human newborn has a preference for human faces. This idea comes from the infant's responsivity to humanness, including the human form and its facial and vocal features. This inborn responsiveness occurs soon after birth and is characterized by the infant's preference to look at human faces and facelike stimuli. This finding was first reported by Robert L. Fantz[15] as early as 1964 but subsequently was repudiated by him because he did not control for the complexity problem. Human faces are more complex than geometric forms. When complexity was controlled, interest in faces was no stronger than interest in other stimuli. Even though we know that there is no inborn preference for the human form, this finding has found its way into textbooks on development. Children do not possess a preference for social forms but may develop one as a consequence of interacting with the various people around them, including parents, siblings, and others. We believe the original finding to be true, although it is false, because it fits with our belief in traits or inborn characteristics of infants that mediate the early mother–child relationship and show that the child has the capacity to form such a relationship from the beginning of life.

Crying Responsivity

By the late 1960s the notion of a responsive mother as a cause of appropriate social development had become well fixed.[16] A responsive mother was characterized as one who responded to her infant's crying, which was good for the child since it made the child feel competent and loved.[17] Benjamin Spock, in the earlier editions of his book *Baby and Child Care*, had argued against responding to infants' crying, especially at night, because it could reinforce the cry and spoil the child—even increasing the child's crying. The new argument was that the maternal responsivity would instead satisfy the child's basic need for interaction; as a result, reinforcing the child's cry by responding to it would lead not to more crying but to less. These two very different ideas—responsivity would be either good or bad for the child's development—set the stage for a study that would show the outcomes of maternal response to infant crying. Bell and Ainsworth[18] obliged with a study comparing maternal responsivity toward infant crying in the first three months of life to infants' crying behavior at the end of the first year. The authors concluded that a mother's responsivity to her infant's crying did not lead to more crying behavior but instead to more communicative behavior.

This study confirmed the belief that maternal responsivity would have positive consequences, and if there was a single study that changed our style of responding to children's crying, it was this one. Ironically, although this study was widely referenced, it has been subject to serious criticism.[19] In fact, the design and analysis of the study do not allow us to conclude that responsivity to crying reduces crying. Even though the new findings that pointed out the errors were reported in a leading journal, the original findings continue to be used—because they fit the commonly held belief that responsive mothering produces socially healthy infants.* Responding to infants' cries may be good for them, but there is no good evidence to support this belief.

---

*It should be noted that prior to the time when responsivity was believed to be best for infants, at least for the first three months of life, other socializing techniques were used. It was thought, for example, that infant crying was good for babies and exercised their lungs.[20]

Milk versus Touch

Harry Harlow, in one of his widely known studies, gave baby monkeys the choice of two inanimate surrogate mother objects. One was made out of wire and delivered milk using a nursing bottle; the other was a cloth mother that did not deliver milk. Harlow reported that baby monkeys preferred physical contact to milk delivery and thus helped set the stage for our belief that children need social/physical contact with their mothers. What is not mentioned in most of the textbooks is that the wire surrogate mothers were cold. The baby monkey chose the cloth mother rather than the wire mother delivering milk because the wire did not retain heat.[21] When the wires were warmed, the monkeys showed no difference in preference between the wire and cloth mothers. This should not be surprising in light of the well-known fact that thermal regulation is a very important task for infants and much of physical contact with mothers has to do with staying warm. We hold to the idea of the importance of physical contact since it supports our belief that young infants (monkeys and humans) need contact with their mothers. Feeding is not the most important role mothers perform; physical contact is.

Motherless Monkeys

Harry Harlow's best-known studies, mentioned earlier, have to do with motherless monkeys.[22] These studies stand as the best demonstration of the effect of lack of early mothering experience on children's subsequent peer and psychosexual development. Harlow demonstrated that children (monkeys) raised without their mothers showed severe problems as adults: difficulty engaging in sexual reproductive acts and, once the female became pregnant, inadequate mothering. Many of these motherless monkeys were abusive and even killed their children. It appears that the role of mothering in one generation affected children's social behavior, including peer interactions and parenting, in the next. There are, however, several very important problems with these studies. To begin with, the motherless monkeys were deprived of all social experiences, not only those with their mothers. It would be difficult to conclude that the effects observed in adulthood were caused by the lack of mothering rather than the lack of any social contact. In fact, when motherless monkeys are raised together, we find that these monkeys do just fine.[23]

Even more critical, however, is the fact that these motherless mon-keys behaved quite differently, and much better, toward their second children than toward their first.[24] If poor or no mothering experience led to poor mothering behavior in the next generation, as the results showed, then some sort of trait must have been formed: poor mothering led to trait X. How then did these motherless monkeys lose the trait X after they had their first child? Trait X should have affected all children they raised. The evidence suggests that their mothering behavior was not fixed by their early lack of mothering experience. Even if the major effect of being raised in isolation was the lack of mothering experience, the motherless monkeys were not permanently abusive and did not remain bad mothers. Something counts besides early childhood experiences!

Institutionalized Children

In the 1940s and 1950s investigators like René Spitz and J. McVicker Hunt found that children being raised in institutions had profound delays in development.[25] Spitz coined the terms *anaclitic depression* and *hospital-ism* to mark what he saw in these children, whom he thought had suffered due to maternal deprivation. The work of Spitz and others on institution-alized children seems to confirm the belief that mothers are important to children's healthy development. However, by the early 1960s there was ample evidence that the developmental retardation in these children was due not so much to lack of mothering as to lack of significant care by anyone.[26] Much as in the Harlow studies, institutionalized children were deprived of all social contact, not only contact with their mothers, and it was difficult to separate these two effects. These findings were con-firmed in a study on institutionalized children done in 1962 by Sally Provence and Rose Lipton,[27] who found that the children in institutions not only were without mothers but were not receiving proper care. For example, the hospitals were understaffed, the workers underpaid and undereducated. They were able to perform only the most elementary tasks, such as feeding (often with the bottle propped up) and changing diapers.

The deprivation argument pitting the loss of mothers against poor social environments remains a critical problem. It is likely that children who are without mothers go without proper social interaction in general. The studies cited convince me that it is the lack of proper social contact, rather than the lack of mothers, that is the deciding force in their poor developmental history.

Child Abuse

Unfortunately, child abuse in our society gives us a good human model through which to explore the effects of poor mother–child experience. Most people believe the widespread reports that children who are abused by their mothers will become abusing parents themselves, despite the fact that the studies that report such findings are retrospective in nature and thus not entirely reliable. To gather data on this topic, abused children are identified in clinics, where information on their parents' childhood experiences is gathered. As reported, their parents are often found to have been abused as children, and so a cause-and-effect connection is made. However, without data on the set of children who are *not* abused but who have parents who were abused as children, it is most difficult to determine the effect of the abuse in one generation on abuse in the next. Many of the people in my generation were physically punished by their parents, yet they are unlikely to punish their children. Stress factors such as poverty and culture, as well as historic changes, have as much to do with how parents behave as do traits of parents themselves.

The recent work on child abuse suggests that the reported link between early negative mothering and subsequent child disturbance is not certain. Dante Cicchetti,[28] in his work with abused children, reports that there are significant numbers of abused and neglected children who are at the same time securely attached; that is, they have a positive relationship with their mothers even though they are being abused by them. This finding and others like it raise questions about how the nature of the mother–child relationship impacts on the child's later mental health.

Current beliefs about how the early mother–infant relationship affects subsequent social adjustment can be seen in the six groups of findings just discussed. As we have seen, these beliefs are often based on false information, yet they persist because the mother–infant relationship is so important to maintaining the traditional organismic model of development. The idea that the mother–child relationship is paramount supports the proposition that what happens early affects what happens later and that development is gradual and continuous. To raise questions about these studies is to raise questions about the theory they are supposed to support.

In place of that theory I have proposed a contextual model, which rests on the central premise that social behavior is determined and controlled by the social structure. When the structure is different, social behavior is different. This broad view of social development allows for the consideration of cultural and individual differences as well as age changes as a function in part of the differences in social environments. Moreover, it allows us to consider the multiple and complex relationships that children can have. Because of this complexity, it becomes necessary to worry about how children's cognitive ability affects and supports complex and multiple social relationships, a problem not raised when only the child's relationship with the mother is considered. Finally, and perhaps most important, it means that our early relationships do not fix our fate. New social structures and supports can and do alter our histories.

ON THE NATURE OF RELATIONSHIPS

The social space of children is made of a potentially large number of social objects—inanimate objects, such as security blankets and toys, as well as animate objects including animals and a wide range of people. It seems clear therefore that all possible relationships in children's social space must be considered in deriving a model of social development. Yet attachment theory discounts all but a specific category of relationships and largely all but one specific person in the child's development. Consequently most other relationships have not been studied to any productive extent.

During our lives we all have love, friendship, and acquaintance relationships, each with a set of rules governing our actions and goals and each associated with different kinds of feelings. Within these broad categories relationships vary and are quite complex, and not all of them can be neatly categorized as attachment or nonattachment—at least not while shedding any light on the role they might play in children's adaptation to their social world. Considering that there is ample evidence that infants and young children are able to establish all three major types of relationships, it is obvious that the developmental sequence and the interconnection among these relationships must be studied.

Some love relationships can be classified as attachment relationships—that is, they provide a secure base—but since it is not clear that a secure base is a necessary part of all love relationships, not all can be categorized this way. That does not mean they have no impact. For example, parents love their children, but children do not necessarily offer a secure base for parents. Love relationships also can be divided in terms of their amount of sexuality. In some love relationships sexuality plays an important role, such as with a spouse, while in others, such as with mothers, fathers, and children, sexuality is normally absent. The dimension of a secure base, or what is called an attachment, and the presence or absence of sexuality form a complex structure that includes a variety of different love relationships, all of which exist in adult experience. Whether such a complex set of love relationships exists for children is unknown. Although a role for sexuality during childhood has been suggested by Freud, it is difficult to study.* Nonetheless, children can and probably do have strong love relationships that both have and do not have a secure base as their primary focus. For example, children love both their parents and their siblings, but they probably are attached only to the former and not to the latter, especially if the sibling is younger than they are.

Friendship relationships are different from love relationships, although the distinction may be difficult to describe. Friendships also vary along different dimensions and at times may merge with love relationships. Like love, friendship may or may not involve sexual behavior. Friendships tend to vary with the age of the participants. They may involve same-age peers, or they may exist between older and younger persons, such as between a day-care teacher and a child. Like love, friendship relationships can be enduring and can exist even without extended interactions.

Acquaintances are those relationships that tend to be the least enduring and the most specific to the particular types of interactions that bring them into existence. They usually occur as a consequence of a particular and highly structured social exchange, such as with a storekeeper or office worker. These relationships vary along a dimension of familiarity, from those in which the members recognize one another,

---

*Childhood sexuality remains a difficult topic to study largely for political reasons. Schools and parents are reluctant to allow surveys and research in this area. What we know is that children are sexual at very early ages—in the United States the average age for first sexual intercourse is fourteen to fifteen, and it is common to find twelve-year-old girls who are pregnant.

know each other's names, and exchange information, such as between employers and employees, to those less familiar interactions as between a shop owner and a customer or with people whom we greet casually, passing them on the street.

There is a fourth kind of social contact, and that is our interactions with strangers. These interactions are particularly important, especially for young children, who by the age of eight months often show very distinct patterns of behavior toward people who are not familiar.* The term *stranger anxiety* has been applied to this period of development to mark the infant's response to strangers. Strangers are, by definition, those people with whom we have no relationship and who are unfamiliar to us. Yet even in this category of nonrelationships there are variations that may be of some importance to our understanding of the young child's broad social network and cognitive ability. For example, strangers who possess particular characteristics may elicit different reactions from strangers without those characteristics. Thus strangers of the same sex or racial background as the child are likely to evoke different reactions from strangers of the opposite sex or of other racial backgrounds.[30]

In the study of children's social development the full array of possible relationships has not been explored or even considered. In part this is due to overwhelming support for the idea that a child's primary relationship is with the mother and all others either do not exist or are unimportant. For any complete understanding of children's social development, we need to trace the development of these other relationships as well, preferably from the children's earliest social interactions. It is clear to me that a complex array of relationships exists early in the life of children and that without delineating the full range of these relationships an exploration of the development of any theory explaining it is incomplete.

If we believe that children can have multiple relationships, then we need to take into account children's cognitive development in any attempt to understand social development. Elaborate networks of people require sophisticated cognitive capacities to keep track of them. Children in the first few years of life are capable of elaborate symbolic operations,

---

*Stranger anxiety is a widely studied phenomenon. Some children show stranger anxiety as early as three months, and not all children show the response. In addition, there is sufficient evidence to suggest that infants in day care show less stranger anxiety than home-reared children.[29]

at least at some level, and have sufficient memory to process information concerning themselves, other people, and the relationships among them. No theory of social development that ignores the cognitive processes of children can be adequate. While space does not permit an exhaustive discussion of these cognitive processes, it is important to note that they support the underpinnings of an elaborate and complex social network. In fact, it has been argued that the complex social network itself, from an evolutionary–adaptive perspective, required and therefore played an important role in the selection of brains capable of abstraction and symbolic representation.

Children could develop according to attachment theory without the elaborate cognitive capacities they have; a simple biologically based, noncognitive model would be sufficient. There is ample evidence, however, that children have cognitive information relative to their social life. They have knowledge of age and sex differences and recognize the familiar; they recognize and respond differentially to boys and girls and to men and women, as well as to age differences.[31] Moreover, infants can differentiate familiar from strange. Elsewhere I have elaborated on children's understanding of themselves and the nature of themselves in relationship to other people.[32] A mother is highly familiar, female, and adult, whereas a father is highly familiar, male, and adult. One's younger sister, on the other hand, is familiar, female, and young. Given children's cognitive capacities, it would be possible for them to construct a coherent map of the social objects in their world.

To look at infants' knowledge about the social world they inhabit, my colleagues and I conducted a series of studies on what we called "social knowledge." In one study we had adults, children, and a small adult (midget), one at a time, approach an infant, who was seated next to her mother in a laboratory room. This procedure, having a person move slowly toward the child without talking and with a frozen smile on the face, is the one used to observe infants' response to strangers. More often than not, from eight or nine months on infants show either concern at the approaching stranger or outright anxiety, including crying. What we hoped to show was that for infants the nature of the stranger would help determine the response and would tell us what the infant was "thinking." As expected, strange adults elicited the most concern and anxiety. The five-year-old children who approached the infants elicited little or no anxiety; if anything, they received smiles and signs of interest. To begin with, then, it was clear that infants could discriminate between them and were more frightened of adults than children. Two features that might capture their attention were the height difference and the round child face versus the elongated adult face. That is where the midget came into the study. If the infants were frightened of tall people, they would show no fear and might smile at the midget (short adult vs. tall adult); but if it were facial features, then they would show fear of the midget, as they did with the adult. The infants showed neither fear nor joy but rather surprise. The infants' surprise suggests that the infants recognized that a person of such a height does not have such an adult apportioned head. While we do not know from this study whether height is more important than facial features, we do know that by eight months infants have a fairly good idea of what people of all ages look like, and, more important, their emotional and social responses are determined by this knowledge.[33] As can be observed in public places, infants and young children often seem more frightened of strange adults than of strange children, and they are more readily able to approach the latter than the former. Whatever form our ideas about socialization may take—maternal attachment theory or systems perspective—we will need to include what children know.

THE SOCIAL NETWORK MODEL OF DEVELOPMENT

The contextual model rests on the idea that the causes of social behavior and development are to be found in the current structure of the social system itself. When the system is altered, behavior and relationships change. An example of the interplay between an individual's behavior and a social system underscores its importance. In research conducted in the early 1960s, Leonard A. Rosenblum studied bonnet and pigtail macaque monkeys.[34] Bonnet macaques cluster together in matriarchal groups so that a mother, her sisters, her adult daughters, and their babies might all be found closely huddled. The pigtail macaques are much more isolated. There are no groups, just the adult female and her baby. The bonnet baby interacts daily and forms relationships with mother, aunt, grandmother, cousins, and siblings, while the pigtail baby interacts and forms a relationship only with its mother. When separated from its mother, the pigtail baby at first shows extreme distress. This is followed by a state of depression. The bonnet baby shows a markedly different pattern. It, too, is distressed by the withdrawal of the mother. However, it soon recovers, using the familiar others who adopt it for its social and affective support. This study demonstrates the power of the contextual approach. In a network where there is only the mother, her loss consti- tutes an enormously significant event, one from which the infant is not likely to recover. In John Bowlby's terms the loss of the mother is a life-threatening event. In a context where there are other significant people, the loss of the mother, while perhaps significant, is not life threatening. Similar findings have been reported when human infants are studied in adoption situations.[35]

In a network where there is *only* the mother as caregiver, the child's first and only relationship will be with her, and the child's other relation- ships must be sequential to and dependent on the first. This sequential deterministic feature, the hallmark of attachment, does not have to be, as some have argued, a biological necessity for the species. Rather it is a feature of the social structure. There is little support for the idea that the social network of humans consists solely of the infant and mother. This idea is not biologically necessary, nor is it historically, culturally, or evolutionarily accurate. Some cultures promote the use of multiple caregivers in the form of mother, female sibling, grandmother, and friends. Some support day-care settings with a few adults and several children, while others support the mother alone with her infant. Mothers are never the only people who interact with infants; others, including fathers, siblings, friends and peers, and other adults, are in continuous contact.[36]

In the last decade there has been an increase in the study of the role of fathers and siblings. The importance of fathers in the play life of their children has now been clearly shown, and we have seen that siblings are important teachers.[37] Although a growing number of studies bear witness to the role of others in children's early development, there are relatively few theoretical perspectives that can be used to anchor the new empirical findings. A social systems perspective is needed—one that takes the view that the child has a place in a broad social network rather than in a unique and specific dyadic relationship. In describing the social network of children, I have suggested that the role of any single relationship cannot be fully appreciated without the broader perspective of placing it into the larger framework of people in the child's life. For example, when the role of the father is considered, an obvious part of the father's role is his interaction with his child. However, he also has an indirect influence; that is, his relationship with his wife, the child's mother, affects how she behaves toward the child. A husband who respects, loves, and supports his wife also supports her interactions with the child. These interactions are likely to be very different from those of the wife without positive support. Single parenthood loses the support—emotional and financial—of a significant other.

By focusing our interest on social systems, we can avoid some of the fallacies of attachment and general organismic models. I see a contextual model as a broader theory, one that can readily incorporate the important ideas of attachment. The most important features of the social systems model are its emphasis on the multiple nature of the infant's early social relationships and its emphasis on the effect of the social environment in determining current adjustment. What we need is a social systems theory that emphasizes current adaptation to the context in which people live. Such an approach has enormous implications for such social policy issues as child day care, family structure, and the role of men and women in a modern society.

The Elements of the System

As soon as we recognize that others besides the mother play at least some role in the child's development, we have to concern ourselves with how the multiple elements in this system are related to one another. The elements within the family include each individual as well as all possible combinations. So, for example, in a family of two children and a mother and father, there are four single elements, six dyads, four triads, and one quadrad. Each one is an element, and the shifting of the individual members is part of the dynamics of the system. The complexity of the set of elements increases as soon as we start to add grandparents, uncles and aunts, cousins, teachers, and peers. It is to this complex network that the child adapts. For some children the network is very small and may include just the mother. But this is a rare event; for most children in our culture the nexus is a complex set of elements.[*]

---

[*]In a recent study[38] we collected data on the social networks of more than one hundred three-year-old children living in the Princeton–Trenton, New Jersey, area, all from intact families. Children in our sample had approximately six friends in addition to a mother, a father, and siblings. The children came in contact with an average of almost ten relatives, including grandparents, aunts, uncles, and cousins, in a month, while the number of adults other than family was approximately seven. On the average, approximately three relatives, four friends, and four adults other than the parents were seen by the children once a week. Such data as these point to the fact that certainly by three years of age children are embedded in a rich and varied social system containing many elements.

The process of gathering data on the significant others is slow. Perhaps we have the most information on fathers and siblings, but much of this work has been reviewed in several books,[39] so suffice it to say that infants do form attachments with their fathers as well as their mothers.[40] We all know this. The role of the father changes as the child gets older and caregiving activities give way to play and education, but even in infancy fathers play an important role.

Children also form relationships with their siblings, and in many cases older siblings play a critical role in a child's development. Judy Dunn[41] has found a powerful and significant effect of siblings even among very young children. Grandparents almost never are considered, which is surprising given that parents of parents exert a strong influence on children's development, if for no other reason than that they influence the child's parents. Even the word *grandparent* should make it obvious that such a role carries with it importance for both child and grandparents.

If the grandparents have been neglected in studies, aunts, uncles, and cousins have simply not been considered. There is almost no information about them. Within the anthropology and animal behavior literature, however, the role of these others is well recognized. In lion prides, for example, the social structure of the group includes the female relatives—mothers, aunts, daughters, and cousins. While the role of the father's brother and mother's brother has been recognized by anthropologists, especially if the father dies, psychological study has been absent.

Peers constitute an important element in children's social systems, all the more so now that more than sixty percent of American mothers of children under the age of three work outside the home. Even in the first two years of life children form relationships and are unhappy at their loss.[42] Peers are good for play and as a model for a child's behavior, since they share equal or nearly equal abilities and are most like the child. They also are good for teaching, especially if they are somewhat older, since their abilities do not differ too markedly from the child's. Peers also protect one another and, most important, are capable of forming strong emotional ties to each other.

Most relevant for our consideration in the 1990s are the relationships of children with teachers, day-care personnel, and babysitters. Even within the first few months infants are exposed to unrelated adults who care for children while parents are away. Given the increasing number of mothers who work outside the home and the changing family structure in the United States, there is increasing child care by unrelated adults. There is little information about children's relationships with these people, although it is clear that positive attachments are formed.[43]

In short, there are many and diverse elements to the child's social nexus, and the constraints on these relationships rest on the nature of the family, which in turn is related to cultural factors.

Interconnection of Elements

Not only is the system characterized by many elements, but these elements are continuously influencing each other. Within the family the interaction of elements can occur at several levels. At the simplest level the infant can affect the parents as the parents can affect the infant and the parents can affect each other, all through direct interactions. When larger units are considered, the interrelation of elements naturally becomes more complex. For example, a child can affect not only each parent separately but also the parents' relationship. Likewise, the father can influence the mother and child individually as well as the mother–child relationship. The mother–father relationship also is likely to affect how the mother behaves toward her child.

The individuals in a social system also can affect each other indirectly, through, for instance, interactions that do not occur in the person's presence. The father's emotional support of the mother, mentioned earlier, is likely to affect the infant. Indirect effects can also occur in the presence of the person, even though that person is not involved in the interaction. For example, Felicia sees that Benjamin is scolded when he draws on the wall of his room. She learns not to draw by watching what happens to him, learning, as a result, that she will be scolded if she does that. All of us learn a great deal by watching what happens to others—we call this *imitation*.

In short, infants adapt to a social system containing elements that vary in number and complexity and that influence the children and are influenced by them, both directly through interactions with the child and indirectly through interactions with each other. Children establish relationships within a network of already existing relationships and, in so doing, create new ones and alter old ones.

Nonadditivity

Systems possess the quality of nonadditivity. This means that knowing everything about the elements that compose the system does not reveal everything about the system and its operation as a whole. Every element or set of elements behaves quite differently within the system than in isolation. Within a family, how an individual person behaves alone can be quite different from how that person behaves in the presence of another. Allison Clarke Stewart[44] observed mothers, fathers, and children in dyadic and triadic interactions and showed that the quality and quantity of behavior between mother and child when alone was changed dramatically when the father joined the group. For example, mothers initiated less talk, played with their children less, and also were less engaging, reinforcing, directive, and responsive to their children when the fathers were present than when they were alone. The child, of course, also exerts influence on the parental relationship. Any couple who has a child knows this. Judy Rosenblatt[45] found that the presence of one or more children reduced parental touching, talking, and smiling. Looking at behavior at the dinner table, we have found that the more children there are, the fewer positive interactions between parents, although the amount of information that parents gave one another did not change.[46] Finally, Ross D. Parke and colleagues[47] found that when mothers were with their husbands, they were more likely to explore the child's body and smile than when they were alone with the child. Moreover, when mothers were with their husbands, they tended to touch their sons more than their daughters, whereas this differ-ence was not evident when the mother and child were alone.

Nonadditivity presents an obstacle in our study of relationships since we would like to believe that the interactions observed between two people remain the same even when more people join the group or when the situation changes. The rule of nonadditivity suggests that this is not the case. The evidence that relations between elements are dependent on the set or subset of elements present suggests the relative nature of our interactions. The dynamics of families and the interactive quality of family members have been the concern of family therapists, the most important group studying these dynamics.

Steady State

Systems maintain themselves at the same time that they change. A steady state is characterized by the interplay of flexibility and stability by which a system endeavors to maintain a viable relationship among its elements and its environment.[48] Social systems are goal oriented, and the steady state principle addresses the need to move toward achieving either different goals or the same goals with changes in the interactions between elements. Within the family such a process appears essential since, by definition, change occurs because of the development of the child. Children's skills, knowledge, and behavior continually change, and this must be accounted for if the family is to maintain itself. The nature of the interaction between the child and the parents alters over the first two years, with the amount of physical contact, especially touching, decreasing, while the amount of looking and talking increases. The maintenance of contact behaviors undergoes change, yet the goal itself remains.

The child's functioning within the family system can be described by adaptation and by the flexibility to develop new behavioral patterns. Both of these are in the service of maintaining the system as goals change. Judy Dunn[49] found that, for first-born children, their independent behavior increased after the birth of a sibling. Although this independent behavior occurred and was encouraged by the mother prior to the birth of the second child and was, for the mother at least, a developmental goal, the amount of, kind of, and opportunity for independent behavior changed as the family system itself changed to include the new member. This consistency in the midst of change has to be an important factor in children's development and adaptation to their social world.

A system such as the family has the task of remaining a family in spite of the dramatic changes that take place over time. The birth of children, their growth and development, and their leaving home all impact on the system. The system is steady state only in terms of the processes that maintain themselves in the face of these dramatic changes. While our analysis specifies the family as the unit under investigation, we might easily consider the same problem for the growth of an individual, especially if we allow for the fact that individuals are made up of changing sets of skills and abilities. The task for the individual, then, is how to maintain self-identity in the face of change.

Goals

All systems are characterized by their purposeful quality. The family system exists to achieve certain goals necessary both to the survival of its members and to the perpetuation of the culture and social order. Families have more specific goals, which include but are not restricted to nurturance. The attachment view of social development not only has restricted the number of significant family members by focusing on the mother but also has limited the types of activities and goals engaged in by the family. If only caregiving/nurturance goals are considered, then it may make some sense to study the mother as the only element of interest. However, other functions in the child's life include play, exploration and learning, protection, social control, and peer skills, which may involve family members other than the mother.[*]

Caregiving goals include feeding and cleaning, at the least, and refer mostly to the biological needs relating to bodily activities. Nurturance goals are the functions of love or attachment. Play goals include activities with no immediate obvious goal, those engaged in for their own sake that may have to do with creativity and learning. Exploration and learning mean finding out about the environment by either watching others, asking for information, or engaging in information acquisition with others. Protection includes care from potential sources of danger, both innate sources, such as falling out of trees or being burned in fires, and others, such as being eaten by a predator, taken by a non-kin, or attacked by another. Social control goals—what we think of as socializing the child, regulating when and how the child eats, sleeps, and so on—represent the restriction of the infant's behavior in the way it can interfere with the behavior of others or for the purpose of teaching specific rules. Peer skill goals include learning how to play with and engage peers, which will facilitate peer relationships later, leading to the production of a new family. I am sure still other goals could also be considered. By understanding the potential list of goals, we can turn our attention to the question, "Who is the best person to deliver these to the child?"

ATTACHMENT OR SOCIAL SYSTEMS IN PRACTICE

In most studies based on attachment theory, the mother–child attachment is determined and compared to a child outcome. *The child's environment at the time of the outcome is rarely observed.* If the child's mother were

---

[*]The study of the functions, needs, and goals of the young child is beyond the scope of this book. To create a list of functions or goals, one could utilize Edward O. Wilson's adaptive functions or Henry Murray's needs functions.[50]

inadequate and produced an insecurely attached one-year-old, why could she not affect the child's subsequent outcomes through continued poor mothering? If we found that, for example, poor peer relations were a function of the child's environment when the peer relations were observed, we could argue for a current environmental or contextual, rather than traitlike, cause of outcomes.

Children adjust to their environments. Infants adjust to their mothers' interactions at each age. If the mother's behavior is consistently poor, the child will be insecurely attached at one year of age and maladjusted at later ages. If the mother's behavior starts out poor but gets better, the child might be insecurely attached at one year but adjusted later, after the mother's behavior has changed. To test this theory, and to understand the role of context in general, we will have to study environments over time in the same detail that we study children and their behavior. The fact that it simply is unfashionable to think of other people in the child's network creates enormous difficulties when the social organization of the society changes and child care ceases to be the sole domain of the mother. The exclusive focus on the mother in attachment theory requires that day-care systems be rejected as developmentally inappropriate for young children in spite of the fact that there is no good long-term support for this position.

There is no reason to believe that, if the child's needs are met, the child cannot develop properly even when not cared for exclusively by the mother. What is critical is that the child's needs be met in the day-care setting. This means finding out what it is that an infant needs, be it, for example, consistent caregiving or educational play. If her needs are met, it may not matter that they are met not by the mother but by some other interested adult. If your child wants to learn to play the piano and you do not play, you make sure you get the best teacher for her, help her focus on her practice, compliment her, etc. It is not necessary for you to do the teaching; it is necessary only to make sure it is done well. The same may be true for child care. But good day care will not be inexpensive if we are to satisfy all of the child's needs.

A social systems approach, addressing the variety of needs important to children's successful adaptation, affords us the opportunity to facilitate development in a more orderly fashion. To do so, however, we must first consider the current goals of the family, society, and child. Then we can focus on meeting each particular goal rather than on trying to foster the early development of a trait from which all else in the future is expected to flow. If successful adult peer adjustment is the goal, we need to study what type of social structure best results in this outcome. Moreover, is this goal reached by earlier relationships with the mother or with others like a good day-care provider, or is this goal best reached by constructing in adulthood social contexts more likely to facilitate it? According to the attachment–organismic model this question would never even be raised, despite a growing body of empirical evidence that it is worthy of exploration.

The problem with the attachment–organismic model is that it tries to explain too much and, in so doing, explains little. The relation between theory and social policy reveals itself here in quite a dramatic fashion. If we approached children's development from a contextual— rather than from an attachment–organismic—point of view, this problem would not occur. The interface between our theories and our practice is nowhere more markedly seen than in this dilemma.

Chapter 10

TIME, SUDDEN CHANGE, AND CATASTROPHE

By the turn of the twentieth century three great voices, each in its own way, had addressed the issue of change. Each argued that change was gradual and that the creation of new forms from old ones most likely accounted for the present characteristics of both the earth and the living creatures on it. Charles Lyell in geology and Charles Darwin in biology both formed their arguments against the prevailing view of creation. The earth and its living creatures did not arise suddenly from God's creation, they argued; rather they developed gradually and continuously. Lyell, for example, believed that "we should [restrict] ourselves to the known or possible operators of existing causes; feeling assured that we have not as yet exhausted the resources which the study of the present course of nature may provide, and therefore, that we are not authorized in the infancy of our science to recur to *extraordinary agents*" [italics added].[1] Darwin, too, rejected the idea of sudden change: "I can entertain no doubt, after the most deliberate study and dispassionate judgement of which I am capable, that the view which most naturalists until recently entertained, and which I formerly entertained, namely that each species has been independently created, is erroneous. I am fully convinced that species are not immutable. . . ."[2] What Lyell did in geology and Darwin did in biology Sigmund Freud did in psychology. His developmental theory rested on the idea that people's lives were organic, continuous, and gradual and that earlier events, especially those with one's parents, affected later ones.

These ideas are at the heart of the concepts of continuity, progress, and gradualism that underlie the organismic model of development. Throughout this book I have challenged this model, pulling it apart and examining each feature to see whether the elements themselves make sense in light of what we now know about change. They do not hold up to scrutiny, nor do the available data support such a model. While I have focused primarily on how the organismic model fits human life, part of the appeal of a model of continuity and predictability rests on the belief that it is useful in other disciplines, such as physics and evolutionary biology. As we shall see in an exploration of time and its relation to the new physics and to evolutionary biology, however, the organismic model does not hold in those fields of science any better than it applies to an individual's life. A replacement for the organismic model of human development must come out of newer theories that have sprung from these fields, theories of catastrophe and complexity.

EINSTEIN'S DREAMS*

There is a place where time stands still. Raindrops hang motionless in air. Pendulums of clocks float mid-swing. Dogs raise their muzzles in silent howls. Pedestrians are frozen on the dusty streets, their legs cocked as if held by strings. The aromas of dates, mangoes, coriander, cumin are suspended in space.

As the traveler approaches this place from any direction, he moves more and more slowly. His heartbeats grow farther apart, his breathing slackens, his temperature drops, his thoughts diminish, until he reaches dead center and stops. For this is the center of time. From this place, time travels outward in concentric circles—at rest at the center, slowly picking up speed at greater diameters.

Who would make pilgrimage to the center of time? Parents with children, and lovers.

Development (like all change) takes place over time; our lives are in time, and so to understand the nature of time is to gain insight into how we think about human development. For some people time moves quickly; for others it drags. Some of us think of time as continuous, others as discontinuous. On the wrists of some the second hand moves continu-

*This heading is taken from Alan Lightman's wonderful book of the same title, as is the quotation that follows.[3]

ously around the circle of hours; for others the second hand moves in discrete units, jerking forward in each quantum of time. Is time continuous or discontinuous? Is its relation to reality absolute or relative? Time seen as discrete and relative challenges our idea of continuity as a reasonable model of human development, so it is important that we understand these dimensions.

The study of time has a long philosophical tradition, starting at least with the Greeks and continuing into the present.[4] Two characteristics that have been considered are continuous versus discrete time and relative versus absolute time. One of the major ways of conceptualizing these problems is to distinguish the idea of time from the awareness of time as Immanuel Kant did when he demonstrated that our notion of time is not a re-creation of time but rather a way of considering it. So, the study of time cannot be a search for "a reality in itself," as Kant put it, a point that must be remembered in any investigation of this subject. Our perceptions of time can be quite different from the notion of time that results from intellectual investigation.

Continuous and Discontinuous Time

From the beginning people noticed the sequential nature of their lives: the seasons passed, the constellations cycled, children were born, people died. From within their bodies they could feel changes, and they could study the orderly progression of them. This they called *time*, and they observed it from both inside the body and beyond it.

The contemplation of time as continuous versus discontinuous, or divisible, has a long history in Western thought. Rather than view time as an independent reality with static properties, Henri Bergson believed that the characterization of time as continuous versus discontinuous occurred within the mind[5]: in our inner selves time is continuous, whereas in our external interactions time is divisible and discontinuous. Three hundred years before Bergson, René Descartes, too, believed that our notion of time has its origin in our inner experiences, the sequences of thoughts and perceptions. Thinking about external events allows us to apply these inner experiences to those events. Stimuli from both inside and outside our bodies lead us to consider time.

But what are time's properties? At first ancient peoples, at least from the writings we have, viewed time as qualitative and phenomenological, a substance of itself, independent of the events that occurred. The ancient Greeks, for example, thought of time as a single entity, such as a cosmological principle or god. Its name was Chronus, and it had human qualities: "And Chronus made out of his own seed fire and wind (or breath) and water."[6] Plato described time as belonging to the world of appearances, or the physical world. It had an idealized existence, similar to the notion of absolute time as developed later by Isaac Newton. But time also had mathematical properties. By the fifth century B.C., the idea of segmented time was mentioned.[7] Subsequently Plato talked of the number of times, suggesting that he considered time a metric that could be associated with numbers.[8] Aristotle elaborated this metric concept, giving time a number and therefore a magnitude or duration.

Time as something living incorporated the concept of continuity; time was an indivisible whole. Time as a metric meant time was not a whole but a series of parts, a quality that was divisible and that could be counted—a discontinuous chain or series. To paraphrase Aristotle, time is a continuous thing because its parts are in succession and touch one another, but it is divisible because it has a magnitude.[9]

The idea that time has the property of both the continuous and the discrete continues to attract us some twenty-four hundred years later, even though most of us think of time as continuous and most of our developmental models depict it as continuous. Perhaps our reluctance to think of time as discontinuous is related to our desire to see ourselves as continuous, a goal made extremely difficult if we believe in a discontinuous time.

The power of the idea of continuous time can be seen in our understanding of clocks. The invention of the timepiece in the sixth century A.D. was based on a very simple principle: what appears to be a continuous energy source, such as a waterfall, gravity, or even sand falling, is divided into units. Because the energy source (the event) is crucial to the existence of the clock, it is difficult for us not to equate time with this thought-to-be-continuous event. The division of time, in contrast, is secondary. In fact how far we divide time appears to be arbitrary, relegating the concept of discontinuous time to a status of lesser credibility. Should the size of the unit be hours, minutes, seconds? Which calendar is correct—Gregorian, Julian, Islamic, or other? In their study of the origins of the universe, cosmologists have begun to ask what the smallest unit of time might be. Though the issue is far from settled, some believe there may be no limit, while others hypothesize that there is a smallest unit, something called a femtosecond, which is 10^{-15} (or one quadrillionth) of a second.

Obviously, to think of time as discrete rather than continuous is difficult, first because it challenges how we view ourselves and second because we have no idea how to measure discrete time. Yet quantum mechanics has forced us to reconsider continuous time. Max Planck and Niels Bohr, among other quantum theorists, informed us that there are quanta of energy change; that is, the electrons of an atom, in particular, do not move in a continuous fashion but rather "jump" from one level to another. If energy is not continuous but jumps in this quantum fashion, time also must jump and therefore must be discrete.[10]

Relative and Absolute Time

We must also view time as either relative or absolute.[11] Relative time can be defined as the overt order of events. It is the most common form our notion of time takes because it corresponds to our own experience with the world. In this sense time is not a thing but the change in things or the movement of things.

Isaac Newton, who formally introduced the concept of absolute time, accepted that time could be both continuous and divisible, without a beginning or an end, but held to the ancient belief that time is not related to events or to the movement of objects but is independent. Time, in this sense, is "physically prior to events."[12] For Newton, "absolute time and mathematical time of itself and from its own nature flows equally, without relation to anything external."[13] Time did not belong to events; events occurred in time, which was absolute or real.

Since it is beyond the scope of this book to explore fully the history of the concept of time, suffice it to say that Newton's notion of time survived until the beginning of the twentieth century. The notion of absolute time, unrelated to events, in particular to the motion of heavenly bodies, was held to be correct until radically altered by modern physics. Through Albert Einstein's revolutionary insight into the nature of relativity, time again was linked inextricably to events; that is, time was considered not absolute but related, as was space, to matter. Rather than being in time, as Newton had averred, events *were* time. Einstein demonstrated that the faster an object moves—and this of course refers to very high speeds—the slower time becomes. Consequently modern physics has ceased to understand time as absolute, indivisible, and unchanging in property.

The idea of time as relative rather than absolute has a direct impact on the formulation of our developmental models. If time is defined as the unraveling of life events, then development—also seen as the unraveling of life events—and time are inseparable, and our ideas about one affect our ideas about the other. The organismic model of development rests on continuity. If time is not continuous, neither is development.

Even though the dominant developmental theories still hold to the idea of absolute and continuous time, the literature abounds with suggestions by those engaged in developmental inquiry that time is relative.[14] One of the best examples comes from Joachim F. Wohlwill, who questioned whether age—that is, time from birth—is synonymous with development.[15] He did so by asking whether age is the independent or dependent variable in the study of developmental processes. By concluding that time from birth does not covary with developmental functions, Wohlwill has led us to believe that the series of events making up a developmental function themselves can be used as the dependent variable and indeed may be better for understanding the independent variables of interest.

Consider the concept of IQ. The use of an IQ score characterized by the ratio of mental ability to age implies that one's place in the series of events and age are not synonymous. That is, if Felicia's IQ is 150, she is advancing along this series of events faster than other people her age, and if Felicia's IQ is 100, she is advancing at the same rate as others. If we ask what is important in terms of how she will perform on some task, it is her mental age rather than her chronological age. Thus we may say that, although she is only four years from birth, Felicia has a mental age of six years.

Another example comes from the study of adolescence, where the onset of puberty rather than age is used as the independent variable.[16] It is change, rather than age or time per se, that must be studied. For example, if we believe that the onset of puberty and the accompanying change in hormonal production influence sexual behavior and interest in dating, then the critical variable to study is not the age of the child but rather the point at which hormonal changes take place. Our overuse of age, time from birth, in most studies of development implies that we continue to view time in a Newtonian fashion—that it is absolute and that events belong in time. Age or time is a continuum on which a series of events can be placed. That this view persists in the face of what we know about time speaks to the power of our Newtonian view.[17]

Newton's idea of absolute time implied that time flows in one direction. In fact, our belief in time as having a unidirectional flow is tied not only to our Newtonian view of the world but also to our perceptual capacities. The unidirectional flow of time allows us to make statements about causality. If one billiard ball starts to move toward another billiard ball that is stationary and strikes that ball and sends it moving, we have no trouble in perceiving and believing that the first billiard ball caused the second to move. A sense of causality is dependent on the idea that time is unidirectional. As Richard P. Feynman so eloquently demonstrated nearly fifty years ago, the notion of causality, and therefore the notion of the unidirectional flow of time, is not necessary in quantum mechanics.[18] Such a concept as this is difficult for us to understand and nearly impossible to appreciate in a world where events are always viewed as occurring in a linear sequence.

If a linear, unidirectional idea of time gives rise to causality, then a nonunidirectional idea breaks it down. This means that earlier events do not have to cause later ones. We can see how this is so in human affairs. A unidirectional view of time does not take into account people's capacity to plan for the future. With consciousness, and with the capacity to conceptualize the future, to make plans and have desires for events yet to happen, people are capable of being influenced not only by past events but also by anticipated events in the future. In a study that can be seen as related to the directionality of time, Klaus Riegel looked at whether behavior among older people was similar five years prior to their death regardless of their age from birth. When he worked backward, rather than forward, in time this way, he found enough similarities to suggest that development may not be entirely unidirectional.[19]

Laura L. Carstensen's study of people's social contact over adulthood and old age revealed similar findings. People alter their behavior by anticipating what their old age will be like. People decide earlier in their lives to alter their social pattern of interaction *prior* to their having to do it because of their old age and infirmity. "The nature and patterns of change [in their social contacts] suggests that people play a volitional role in the reduction. Thus, the motivational basis for age-related changes must be considered."[20] That is, the ability to plan for the future shares with quantum mechanics the suspension of time as a causal agent.

We have been talking about people's notions about time. In addition, we can examine people's psychological awareness of time. When we do so, we find that it is a relative, rather than an absolute, view that predominates. Klaus F. Riegel calls relative time, as I have been using the term, *dialectical time:*

> The dialectical concept of time emphasizes concrete experiences and events. As these lead to the formation of conflicts and resolutions ... temporal markings, produced by the synchronization of these sequences, are generated. These ... represent transitions in the sequences of qualitative changes.... The contrastive comparison between simultaneous spatial conditions and developmental temporal changes elucidates the basic properties of the dialectical concept of time.[21]

Since time is the ordering of events, the problem of the measurement of these events becomes relevant. In some sense, then, dialectical time involves the perceived sequence, the measurement used, and the events being recorded. In Riegel's discussion of historical change or development, we see these forces played out. For him, as for others,[22] history, either of the group or of the individual, is a construction of the actual events, their relation to one another, and how they fit into the perceiver's personal narrative. Riegel's analysis allows us to translate the ideas of relativity and quantum mechanics into a psychology of the awareness of time.

The work on a relative view of time is extensive, and it focuses on personal narratives.[23] Most would agree that general or personal history consists of the construction of a past series of events in a form that makes them a consistent and reasonable narrative. They may be discontinuous; however, the narrative serves to create a continuous chain.[24] The stringing together of these events in our narrative produces variable duration lengths. Riegel gives us an example of this. When subjects are asked to recall the people influential in political and governmental affairs, they name people in such a way as to suggest that they view history as a progression of catastrophes, wars in particular.[25] This construction of the sequence of events is relative, and because wars do not occur over fixed time periods, the duration between events, or the memory of the duration, varies widely.

These studies of narrative give rise to the notion that equal units of time (as in months or years) do not represent general units in the process of development.[26] This appears to be true across the entire life course. Children's memory for displaced objects remains the same between birth and six months of age, but between the ages of six and eight months infants start to search for a missing object when it is hidden under another object.[27] From a process point of view, zero to six months represents one unit of time and six to eight months another. There is no reason, therefore, to divide time into equal units. There are two events: no search with a duration of six months and search with a duration of the rest of the life span.

When we divide time into months or years, we accept the idea that development takes place within time rather than being time. By reconstructing time not as a series of equal units, we may be better able to view the process of change.

If time is relative and duration variable, then the units of time do not remain equal but exist as a variable metric—a relativistic view of time that proves to be widely applicable. Look at how age perception varies as a function of the observer's age. At twenty-five years of age Benjamin has no trouble discriminating eighteen- to thirty-year-olds but is unable to differentiate the faces of forty-five- to seventy-five-year-olds. His father, who is sixty years old, on the other hand, has no trouble discriminating the forty-five- to seventy-five-year-olds but cannot discriminate the eighteen- to thirty-year-olds. The observer's judgment about another's age varies as a function of the observer's age.[28]

Age usually is divided into equal time periods, for example, months or years. We generally think there are as many units between fifteen and thirty years as between forty-five and sixty. The analogy is a ruler with equal units. However, this equal metric is not equal for all of us, nor is it unequal in the same way for different ages. Like the observers in the study of relativity, time changes for one but not the other. This, as well as similar findings reported by others, gives rise to the inescapable conclusion that our awareness of time is relational.[29] Yet our methodology for studying development for the most part remains compatible with the notion of time as absolute and connected.

The Connectedness of Time

Of even more importance for any theory in which earlier events are thought to determine later ones is the idea of the connectedness of time. Causality requires a connection between two temporally related events. In spite of the common error that if one event follows another in time they necessarily are causally related—*post hoc, ergo propter hoc*—this belief provides the basic framework of behaviorism. Even if we were to accept the idea of connectedness, we have to be aware of the fact that, as the time between two events increases, the level of connectedness appears to decrease. In almost all empirical research that attempts to relate events over time, the correlation between two events decreases as the time between them increases. Thus events A, B, C, and D in general are likely to follow a simplex pattern: A is most correlated to B, then to C, then to D; and B is most correlated to C, then to D. Duration of time and the association of events in time do not readily support the belief in connectedness. Of course, such findings mean that our idea of primacy—that what happens in the early part of our lives affects us forever—may be wrong as well.

The interval between events also affects our demonstration of continuity. For example, we assume discontinuity in a butterfly's development from the sequence of larva to caterpillar to butterfly because the interval from A to B and B to C is too large. If our observations were increased so that very short intervals and many observations were taken, we might be able to observe the morphology of a single cell of the butterfly and then conclude that there is more continuity than we originally thought. On the other hand, were there too short an interval between events A and B, we also might not be able to observe continuity. Consider the property *liquid*. A liquid is the movement of molecules, a movement that appears continuous. Actually, however, it is a sequence of discontinuous events. Filming with a high-speed camera and a microscope, we could observe the movement of these molecules but we would not observe a liquid as such. To observe liquids, we need longer intervals between points. The property liquid thus is interval dependent. If time is continuous, then continuity can be demonstrated only as a function of measurement, in particular the measurement of the interval between points A and B. If continuity can be established only by very short intervals between events, and larger intervals show no connectedness, continuity will do us little good in a predictive science of behavior. It is only by allowing us to predict over relatively long intervals that a developmental approach serves us. Being able to predict only five minutes ahead is not predicting development, only moment-to-moment change.

If Newtonian physics provided the basis of causality as related to temporal relations, then quantum mechanics provides the basis for its rejection. Quantum mechanics makes no assumption about causality. Physics may have little to do with psychology, and the laws of physics may not be relevant to the laws of psychology. Nevertheless, I will assume there are general laws that inform all aspects of human inquiry. In such a view the lack of continuity is not an issue of measurement duration or of measurement error but a property of time. If there is no causal overlapping of events, as there is in Aristotelian or Newtonian physics, predicting events over time may not be possible.[30]

In summary, we tend to think of time as a continuous process, an uninterrupted flow, as Aristotle believed, events touching on one another. This view, carried forward into modern science by Newton, has been replaced by the postclassical physics of the twentieth century, by relativity, which demonstrated first that time was not absolute and second that time was a property of events. This new insight strongly altered the Newtonian view of time, but it was for quantum mechanics to settle the issue of continuity and discontinuity. The new physics has much to teach those interested in development and the relation of time to development. The world view offered by quantum mechanics makes it clear that time, a property of events, cannot be continuous since nature "jumps" and therefore events cannot touch one another. It also calls into question our belief in continuous human development.

NATURE DOES NOT MAKE LEAPS
(NATURA NON FACIT SALTUM)

If time at the level of a human life is not continuous, then at the level of species we may not find continuity either. In fact we do not. Nowhere is the ideal of gradual and continuous change better served than in the theory of the evolution of life. Charles Darwin's theory of evolution explained the historical change in life through the use of natural selection. Although warned by his friend T. H. Huxley that his idea of gradualism was neither necessary nor easily defensible, Darwin, taking his lead from Charles Lyell's theories of geological change, held that change occurs gradually and that new forms emerge slowly from old ones. It is not surprising that he took such a position, because it conflicted with that of the creationists and clearly marked the difference between his view and theirs.

Darwin was wedded to the theory of gradualism as captured in the Latin phrase attributed to Linnaeus—*natura non facit saltum*, nature does not make leaps. Darwin's commitment to gradualism, however, do not invalidate his ideas of random mutation and current adaptation as the bases of change. Nevertheless, gradualism did suggest, at least for many who followed Darwin, an organismic model since continuity and gradual change remain at its heart. Gradualism in evolution implies first that the fossil record for the origin of new species should consist of a sequence of continuous and sensibly graded intermediate forms linking the descendant to its ancestors and second that if there are morphological breaks in a postulated phylogenetic sequence these should be due to imperfections in the geological record.[31] Yet a theory of gradualism, as opposed to a theory of natural selection, cannot be defended using the evidence available.[*] Stephen Jay Gould, addressing the imperfections in the geological record, stated, "The extreme rarity of transitional forms in the fossil record persists as the trade secret of paleontology. The evolutionary trees that adorn our textbooks have data only at the tips and nodes of their branches; the rest is inference, however reasonable, not the evidence of fossils."[33]

Gould and his colleague Niles Eldredge, over twenty years ago, offered a theory that the evolution of species involves stasis, a period of predictable change during which the laws of natural selection appear to work gradually, and sudden appearance, periods when species appear (or disappear) relatively suddenly and fully formed.[34] This theory is now supported by a large set of evidence.

Recent developments in the understanding of our evolutionary past support the idea of sudden change. To begin with, the fossil record shows a burst of animal evolution in the Cambrian period, over 550 million years ago. It was, as we now can see, the greatest burst of evolution the planet has ever known: "The lid was off; evolution was going full tilt. Never again in the history of marine life do we see so many phyla, classes, or orders appearing so rapidly."[35] This certainly is no support for gradualism. The evidence for the creation of life is filled with such bursts, and so is the fossil evidence for extinction. Almost a decade ago, David M.

---

[*]There is little argument that natural selection can occur quite rapidly. Jeffrey S. Levington argues that even unmatched bursts of creativity in the production of new species seen six hundred million years ago can readily be explained by natural selection. In fact he shows how rapidly natural selection can act, focusing on James A. Grant's work on finches. Levington states, "An intense dry spell killed all the plants except those with large drought resistant seeds. Because the finches are mainly seed-eaters, their mortality was high. These circumstances favored an increase in the average beak size, because birds with larger beaks could crack open large seeds. As Grant observed, fluctuations between dry and wet conditions caused continuous bouts of evolution, often in the span of just a few months."[32]

Raup explored the extinction rates found in the record.[36] Rather than show a continuous pattern, they showed periods of sudden death, such as at the end of the Cretaceous period. Raup questions whether, in general, extinction is episodic versus continuous. He concludes that there were five mass extinction periods—Ordovician, Devonian, late Permian, terminal Triassic, and Cretaceous—covering a period from more than five hundred million to sixty-five million years ago. The Permian emerges as the largest extinction period, with estimates of species being killed varying as high as ninety-six percent. These data argue for an episodic rather than continuous extinction process. In fact, Raup has proposed a twenty-six-million-year extinction periodicity.

Perhaps the best and most widely known sudden change involves the extinction of the dinosaurs. We are now probably all familiar with the theory put forth by Luis W. Alvarez[37] that the impact of an asteroid with the earth led to the loss of light and vegetation and, with it, the speedy death of many species, including the class of dinosaurs. Alvarez's theory initially met with considerable skepticism, but it now is widely accepted as valid. It should not be forgotten that with the extinction of these large reptiles the earth became more hospitable to other forms, namely mammals, and the rise of the mammalian order and with it humankind became possible. This possibility was the consequence not of gradual change but of a sudden accidental event, the chance encounter of a giant asteroid with the earth. It should be mentioned in passing that the periodicity of extinction and the bursts of new life may be related, in general, to accidents; some have even suggested that the earth periodically comes into contact with meteorites and that the burst of extinction and emergence may be related to these accidents.

Such findings as these contradict the accepted model as offered by Lyell and Darwin. Extinctions for them are randomly distributed in time, and the explanation of the cause of extinctions (or even bursts of new forms) is not to be "found in the alien world of cosmic collisions."[38] Extinction was viewed as a constructive process, where less well-adapted organisms are eliminated and give way to new, and perhaps more successful, species. Raup argues "that extinction, although selective, is not constructive . . . [and] may be just a matter of chance susceptibility of the organism to these rare stresses."[39] The extinction of the dinosaurs, after the dinosaurs had coexisted with mammals for more than a hundred million years, allowed the rise of the mammals. But the dinosaurs did nothing "wrong" in a Darwinian sense; they disappeared through accidental encounter, perhaps a random event. The event, in this case the collision of a large asteroid with the earth, is random to life on earth but may not be truly random. As some have suggested, there may be a lawful reason why asteroids collide with the earth. Nevertheless, it is random to the development of life on this planet.

Evolutionary theory, characterized as both natural selection and gradualism, along with other, similar ideas about change, became the prototype for a general theory of development that, too, held to gradualism and continuity. The data from evolutionary biology have been used to support that idea of development. But if, as I have tried to show, evolutionary biology has rejected gradualism, we should be prepared to consider that human lives are filled with both stasis and sudden change. This requires only that we reconsider the existing data in light of the new world view. A closer examination will reveal, for example, that human growth, viewed as a continuous process that changes its velocity with age, is instead a discontinuous, periodic process of saltatory spurts. To quote Michel Lampl and colleagues, who recently studied children's growth patterns, "90 to 95 percent of normal development during infancy is growth-free and length accretion is a distinctly saltatory process of incremental bursts punctuating background stasis."[40] I suggest that closer investigation of many of our growth functions will reveal similar findings. Robert B. McCall's data on consistency in mental ability over the first two years of life is an example in another domain of change. He demonstrates, at least in a prediction sense, periods of consistency followed by transitions followed by periods of consistency in children's mental development.[41] This pattern of sudden change punctuating stasis is likely to be a more useful model for explaining both human development and such diverse topics as the evolution of life and geological and weather features.*

If we reject gradualism and continuity in evolutionary development and in physics, there may be little reason to retain it for individual development. In its place we may have to consider models that incorporate discontinuity and learn what they reveal about the nature of change.

---

*Weather patterns have now been found to change rapidly with the onset of cold periods being more sudden than had been thought.[42]

CATASTROPHE

The organismic model, which rests on a particular view of time and the nature of the physical universe, when applied to either human lives or the development of species, finds little support. What then might we look toward to study human behavior? Since predictability from past events is not possible, I have proposed that a contextual or pragmatic model be adopted in place of the organismic model. Random events, chance encounters, accidents, and consciousness all stand between past and present. We all witness this chaos in our own lives and those of others. Anyone who has ever attended a class reunion comes away with this surprise: the class leader who was expected to do great things ended up with a life of failure, and the quiet classmate never considered especially bright ended up as a college professor.

The unpredictability of human lives is undeniable. We see it, for example, in the Quiz Kids, the children selected in the 1940s and 1950s for the radio and TV show of the same name because of their brightness, few of whom ended up being very successful intellectually.[43] A recent review of Edward O. Wilson's autobiography also reflects the limits of our ability to predict:

> Wilson was born in Alabama into a family that had never included a scientist or an academic, or even a college graduate. He was the only child of parents who divorced when he was seven, leaving him in the care of others. His father degenerated into alcoholism and eventually committed suicide. His formal education began at seven at a military boarding school and continued through a succession of fourteen schools, in and out of Alabama, during the next eleven years. Wilson grew up in one of the most racist and segregated parts of America, where one's highest aspiration was to become an officer in the military and carry on the Confederate spirit. As a child, he suffered from impaired hearing, and in the year of his parents' divorce he became virtually blind in one eye when a spine of a pinfish pierced the pupil of his right eye. He describes himself as chronically poor at mathematics, unable to memorize lines of poetry, and as having difficulty in copying numbers correctly or in visualizing words, spelled out letter by letter. This is not exactly the start one expects for a Harvard University Professor, least of all a biologist renowned for painstaking observations of ants.[44]

From such a background, it is hard to imagine the emergence of a great scientist; more important, it is impossible to predict, as reviewer Jared Diamond states:

> Nothing is so fascinating or complicated as the trajectory of a human life. We emerge partly programmed at birth, and we change with our experiences thereafter. Some of us finally blow apart in adulthood like long-fuse time bombs, while others grow to shine brightly like comets. Most of us have less spectacular careers, *which are still hard to explain in hindsight, even to ourselves, and impossible to foresee in detail* [italics added].[45]

Nevertheless, the idea of a nondeterministic universe is hard for all of us to accept, and many who resist it will say that prediction is difficult or even impossible not because the life course is not deterministic but simply because it is too complex. What this means is that even if there is order in the universe, and therefore in human development, it is a deep order, one that can do us little good in predicting the development of a single person. As such, its application to helping us form an educated and just social policy toward children and families is limited. While we are being forced to such a conclusion, we should look with interest toward the new models that attempt to understand change.

Work in chaos theory suggests that the failure of prediction may be due to the models of change we have considered. Change may not be linear; in fact, there is little likelihood that linearity is a property of the universe. Until recently this dependence on linearity—both in theory and in our mathematical models—has restricted our range of possible explanations. Eldredge and Gould's principle of stasis and sudden change reminds me of the example most used in catastrophe theory, that of the change from water to steam. This change occurs as a sudden leap following the slow accumulation of heat. In catastrophe theory the leap is due to a sudden change in the variable X, caused by higher levels of the variable Y. Water molecules move faster when heated until such a point in the heating process that liquid water turns to steam and takes on the properties of a gas. A similar analysis is possible for cooling water and the change in state of cold water to ice crystals. In these cases the continuation of Y (the removal of heat) suddenly alters the property of X.

Over the last thirty years investigators have evoked at least four principles that explain discontinuous events. The first is called *initial difference*. Using weather models, we now know that two events that appear to be totally different can be derived from very similar events that have initial differences only. Thus what appear as two totally different developmental outcomes start as very similar events. Given the large number of interactions in the course of a life history, small differences can become exaggerated into radical differences as a consequence of the large number of interactions that serve to elaborate the initial difference. The sequence of interactions is not ordered and is often random, so the differences observed could not have been predicted.

Of particular interest for those interested in considering the organization of development is the second principle, called the *reiterative principle*. Here a complex form can be derived from a single form that is repeated again and again. All that is needed to understand what appear to be random forms is the basic form and some reiterative rule.[46] Such a rule allows for the generation of complex forms like seashells. Adding both the first and second principles, we see that any small difference in the original form, through reiteration, will appear at the end as an enormous difference.

One strong principle derived from both evolutionary biology and chaos theory is the belief in a limited number of patterns, forms, or actions.[47] The argument supporting this belief is complex and involves the generation of sequences and forms from a very large database, made possible by high-speed computers. The possibility of a finite number of structures of very complex forms is even stronger when combined with the belief that these finite structures cross accepted taxonomies. Consider two examples of a finite number of structures. In evolutionary biology it has been noticed that the record does not show a large number of random and varied patterns, which would be likely if the principles of natural selection were being followed. For example, natural selection holds that there is a random generation, through mutation, of a variety of forms and that only those forms that selectively fit with the demand of the environment are likely to survive, the others dying out. If this were the case, we might expect to see many diverse sets of random mutations, a small proportion of which would "succeed" in altering the species. Our fossil record should show failed mutations, faces with eyes in the front and back or bodies with two heads. This does not appear to take place, suggesting that there may be some limit to the random generation through mutation of forms. There may be a strong possibility Darwin was wrong and that not all forms or structures are possible.

In terms of structures that cross the accepted taxonomies, many examples are possible. The shape of a jellyfish and the shape made when a drop of water falls into water bear striking similarities; the time between drops of water from a faucet bears a mathematical similarity to the time between cars in a stream of cars passing a fixed point on a highway. That there could be a similarity between such diverse forms suggests that there are *attractors*, forces that restrict the possible and underlie the finite forms that exist.

The last principle is nonlinearity. Using new models, mathematicians have discovered that, while variables may covary in a linear fashion over part of a range of values, there is no reason to assume that they need to covary linearly over the entire range. This is the principle of catastrophe theory as proposed by René Thom and E. C. Zeeman. It allows us one way to model events without relying on gradualism or simple linear notions of causality.[48]

Catastrophe is best explained by the example already given of the change in water. Catastrophe models possess at least some features that have been used to explain development, as well as fitting into a framework of post-Newtonian mechanics. These features include a range of values where continuity can be seen, or what we have called stasis; a sudden transition, or discontinuity, in the area where the change takes place; and divergence, where a small change in one feature may produce radical changes in another. The findings here readily support Eldredge and Gould's notion of stasis and punctuated change.

Such ideas as these have begun to enter into our explanations of development.[49] The term *chaos* would lead us to believe that events are truly random, but those exploring the theory often give the impression that with big enough computers and complex enough programs we might be able, at least some day, to predict many seemingly random future changes successfully. As we have seen, however, quantum mechanics dissuades us from this view. As Robert Poole has stated, chaos theory is related to Newtonian physics:

> Chaos is a type of randomness that appears in certain physical and biological systems, and is intrinsic to the system rather than caused by outside noise or interference. A well known example is the orbit of Pluto. Although the orbits of the other planets in the solar system are mostly regular, Pluto's path is complicated and impossible to predict over the long term. This case arises because Pluto is gravita-

tionally kicked by other planets as it circles the sun resulting in a path so sensitive to deviations that a change of a few feet in its position now could completely change its resulting location in the next several thousand years.[50]

Chaos does not seem to have an explanation in quantum mechanics. As Poole aptly puts it, "If chaos does exist on the quantum level, it raises confusing questions about the meaning of quantum mechanics. If it does not, the result could be even more profound."[51]

In a sense, chaos theory has generated ideas about predictability, not chance. However, as I tried to show earlier, chance and randomness are likely to exist, and any theory of change must be prepared to embrace this fact. Catastrophe theory stands midway between the simple linear and gradual models and those of chance and accidents that I favor.

FIXITY OF BELIEF

Why then do we cling to such beliefs about the fixity of human nature? Cling we do. Given new knowledge and new measurement procedures, we continue to return to our old model. Under pressure to attain "more knowledge" or "better measures," we return to our belief in prediction and control. Take, for example, the recent surge in knowledge about genes. The recognition of what genes are (their structure) and their relation to behavior and function has given rise again to the idea that earlier events cause later ones and that prediction may be possible. The human genome project promises to explain, through the working of the genes, both human behavior and illness.[52]

But the gene story is far from simple. First consider that humans most likely possess between 50,000 and 100,000 genes. While a few diseases, for example, are related to a single gene, most diseases and most of human behavior are related to a combination of genes. The number of possible combinations given 75,000 or so genes is staggering, on the order of 75,000! (factorial)—a number derived by multiplying 75,000 by 74,999 by 74,998, and so on down to 1, yielding a product larger than the number of neurons in the human brain! Moreover, the location or context of the gene relative to other genes on the chromosome affects the gene's expression as does the geometry of the chromosome. Perhaps even more important, there are mutations in the genes themselves that are not there to begin with. These mutations are likely to be random. The mutations and combinatorial factors make it impossible to develop a predictive relation between fixed traits and outcomes. There are no fixed and unalterable patterns to be found easily.[*]

If a deterministic and predictable pattern concerning genes and behavior cannot be identified, it is clear that our ideas about development need to change. I am forced after thirty years to reject the organismic model, and I now accept the idea that chaos and catastrophe exist, that chance encounters and accidents occur. Predictability is unlikely since the task of living organisms, large and small, is to adapt to their current context. We need to return to Darwin's idea that all phenomena are open to random change (although there is likely to be some limit) and to adaptation—some more so than others but all included.

Such a view poses a serious threat to the world view that the developmental process itself is continuous and that earlier events cause later ones. Why, then, have developmental theories and models based on such premises remained largely unscathed? I believe, as I said in Chapter 4, that the reason for this lies in the usefulness of continuity—for our own lives and for our life narratives. Self-identity requires continuity, that we see our lives and those of others around us as a continuous flow. Our idea of time is dependent on our inner sense of ourselves. It is a difficult conception to give up because we are unable and unwilling to relinquish our belief in our own identity, that we are the same even as we grow and age. Nevertheless, such a limited world view must give way to a different concept of time and development, one that relies on quantum mechanics and speaks to the discontinuity between events. Only by doing so can we understand how development works and how we can effect social change.

Besides more complex models, we need to recognize that randomness really does exist and that in our lives no predictable course of development may be possible. Studies of time, evolutionary biology, and catas-

---

[*]Although the possible combinations are astronomical, techniques currently being developed may make the job somewhat easier. They are called quantitative trait loci (QTL) linkage strategies.[53] Flint et al. used this procedure to identify a set of occurring behaviors, emotionality in mice as measured by motor inhibition and defecation, and were able to identify three loci on the murine chromosomes 1, 12, and 15 that appeared related to these behaviors. Even so, the task is dependent on identifying an inherited family set of behavioral dysfunctions, a task of some difficulty since most disorders do not show such a pattern.[54]

trophe theory lead us away from the organismic model of development and toward a new way of thinking about human development. Sudden change, chaos, chance encounters, and random accidents need not leave us feeling ungrounded and fearful. The contextualism of William James, a view that emphasizes the role of current adaptation, presents us with a model that allows for more optimism than has historicism. Our lives are determined by the adaptive necessity of our current contexts. We are not determined by our pasts but can and do alter our fate.

Chapter 11

CURE OR CARE

⸻◦◦◦⸻

My son, Ben, wears glasses. He has worn glasses since the age of five. Before receiving the glasses, he could not see well. When he was given the glasses, he was able to see better. His poor eyesight was made into good eyesight. His ophthalmologist today prescribes lenses to improve his vision *now*, making no assumptions about past or future. Undoubtedly she would say she has not cured his poor eyesight, for as soon as Ben removes his glasses he can no longer see well. Rather, she provides care for his current poor eyesight.

Although this simple example comes from medicine, it illustrates the different types of social policy that can result when we adhere to a contextual rather than an organismic theory of development. Modern American society, dependent as it is on the organismic model, tends to support policies that favor cures rather than care for human needs. To search for a cure for disease—even for poor eyesight—is indeed a noble and good cause. But when so-called curative measures prove again and again to be fruitless, and when the relentless pursuit of cures deters us from providing necessary care, I believe it is time to review our social policies and the model of development that drives them. Care, as applied to social policy, is consistent with the contextual model of development, the model advocated throughout this book.

When I talk about care, I mean doing something now, for the sake of doing it. Care is given now not because of anything that occurred in the past or that may occur in the future but to alleviate the current difficulty. If, as I have argued, the antecedents of the conditions that children and families find themselves in are not readily knowable, and if the long-term consequences of early care also are not knowable, then the care given to people in the present must be based on its current appropriateness or good.

Cure, on the other hand, implies something radically different. It implies an end point, and this dictates certain solutions and rejects others out of hand. It implies that there is a progression and direction to development. Inherent in devising a cure for anything is the ability to predict the future as well as to know the causal factors that produced the condition. But if it is not easy or even possible to know antecedent conditions or to predict what is likely to happen in the future, as I have argued, then why choose cure over care? Throughout the book I have mentioned the impact of our developmental models on social policy. By social policy I mean nothing more than how we treat our children, referring to how parents raise children in families and how we, as a society, see intervening in children's and families' lives to provide care when needed. In this latter case we usually talk about intervention programs that reflect nothing more than the noble attempt to improve the lives of citizens in need.

When we intervene in people's lives, we should expect many different levels of effect, from limited change, in both level and duration, to permanent change. While many areas of intervention do not require permanent change to be considered successful, within social reform and education society often expects and requires it. But permanent change implies that the change takes place in the person rather than in the environment. This criterion for success biases the conclusions that can be reached by requiring the most radical outcome. A true model of cure, one that fits the organismic model of development, is both absolute and permanent. It is an intervention in the present that promises to correct something in the future, that connects past with present or present with future. But these types of cures are indeed few. In the medical field, for example, it turns out that the vast majority of treatments are forms of care, not cure. One type alters behavior of a diseased state for only a brief period. Administering nitroglycerin to a patient with angina temporarily relieves the pain, but of course it does not remedy the cause of the pain or provide long-term relief. It certainly is not a cure in its most stringent form; it is care, something that affects behavior now. Nevertheless, anginal pain is reduced. A second type is prosthetic, such as caring for poor vision with corrective lenses. Here the intervention is absolute but not permanent. Most forms of disease are treated this way: care is achieved through the prosthetic intervention, but the problem is never entirely gone. Hypertension is, for example, controlled successfully through the use of a particular medication and diet. When the intervention is stopped, the hypertension returns.

These few examples point out how elusive a true cure is, even in medicine, where the biological basis of the problems to be addressed might suggest a greater possibility of permanent cure than in social problems, so interwoven with the environment. The examples also show that care at the moment produces change and so imply that care can alter behavior.

What we need to do for children and families in need is to maintain care and not expect it to act as a cure for the future. Turning to social policy, the research on intervention in poor children's lives demonstrates that when they are given special educational opportunities they are capable of utilizing them. Their school performance is significantly better than those of poor children who do not receive the educational intervention, and it matches those of middle-class children.[1] Instead of being pleased with the fact that intervention works and that these children's lives are improved, our policy makers are displeased because of the finding that intervention now does not affect their behavior over time. Within three years of stopping the intervention these children lose most of the educational gains they had made. The conclusion of policy makers is "Why have we spent all this money? There are no long-term benefits." This would be akin to saying, "Well, you have worn glasses for five years. You should be able to see well without them now." Of course, we make no demand that wearing glasses now affects what occurs later, for we know that as long as we maintain the intervention the desired goal is reached. Why, then, is that demand made for educational intervention? It is an absurd requirement, similar to requiring of religion that confession last week, after many years of sinning, last a lifetime. In actuality, in the Catholic Church it is understood that people will need this intervention throughout their lives.

Still another problem in organismic theories is a temporal sense. We do not know when or how good parenting affects children's behavior in the future. Does it affect their peer relationships or their own parenting?[2] Proponents of the organismic theory insist that any intervention affects later behavior. But since we do not know when, or even how, it will affect events later, we are likely to have trouble demonstrating its effectiveness. When, however, we take a contextual, not an organismic, approach, we do not require effectiveness in the future but only effectiveness now.

The belief that what happens at one point in time should impact on another cannot be demonstrated, either in theoretical form or in terms of educational or health needs. Such an expectation of permanence places an unfair burden on social and educational interventions that is rarely, if ever, imposed in other areas of life, such as in health or technology. This requirement for cure grows out of our belief that earlier events do affect later ones and therefore our interventions should seek to affect events both now and later. In Chapter 4 I argued that in fact earlier events do not necessarily affect later ones, so if we wish to effect change, we need to do so without expecting permanent cures or effects in the future. Instead we need to maintain the intervention to achieve and maintain the desired goal. Whether in education or in health, we must commit ourselves to the continuing care of people, regardless of whether that care, once terminated, leads to subsequent behavior. The demonstration that the care has current effectiveness is all that is needed.

TRAITS VERSUS ENVIRONMENT

The medical analogies offered so far have obvious limitations. More than in cases of social ills, it is possible that cures can be found for many diseases. It is quite likely, for example, that someday doctors will be able to perform surgery to correct Ben's poor eyesight and he will no longer need the care of eyeglasses. Even then, of course, changes in his environment as well as the inevitable accidents and chance events might disrupt the permanence of the cure and necessitate further care. There is hope for medical cures because of the biological basis of most disease; that is, Ben's poor vision is apparently a trait that resides in him. Even so, as the discussion of genes in Chapter 10 indicated, such cures may be unattainable for all but a few diseases. Cures become even more elusive as the causes become more complex. Thus they may be totally unavailable in development in general. The organismic model includes the theory that the engine of change and the structures that undergo change reside within the child. This stands in contrast to the contextual model, where the engine of change and the characteristics of children are determined in large part by their current environment.

One good example is the social policy related to aggression in children. In the organismic or trait model the causes of violence are located in the child. Whether violence initially is caused by biological factors such as genes, birth trauma, or low birth weight, or by socialization factors, such as aggressive parents, a characteristic exists within the individual that accounts for it. This organismic or trait model also implies that the child will express violence in the future as a consequence of these internal traits. Thus violence is predicted from earlier events located in the child. Regardless of whether the trait is genetically or socially produced, once the trait has been established it resides in the child and will be expressed later. Our society tends to believe that this model is correct; some believe it because of a belief in the biology of aggression and some because of a belief in environmental causes. But in both cases the cause, however created, resides permanently in the child. There is, however, important counterevidence to suggest that such a model may be inadequate to explain our societal ills. In an excellent review on the cycle of violence, Cathy Spatz Widom points out that

> despite widespread belief that violence begets violence, methodo-
> logical problems substantially restrict knowledge of the long-term
> consequences of childhood victimization. Empirical evidence for
> this cycle of violence has been examined. Findings from a cohort
> study show that being abused or neglected as a child increases one's
> risk for delinquency, adult criminal behavior, and violent criminal
> behavior. However, the majority of abused and neglected children
> do not become delinquent, criminal, or violent.[3]

Many other studies, too, confirm that the trait model explains too little of the outcome.

The contextual model holds that when children live in a context of violence they are more likely to become violent.* Given the fact that many children experience violence on a daily basis, it is no wonder that they have become more aggressive. The best evidence for a contextual basis of violence is the relation between handgun use and murder rates. One study showed that in 1989 the murder rate in Seattle, Washington, was many times higher than that in Vancouver, British Columbia, although the two cities had similar populations, similar climates, and

---

*Of course, there are individual differences here too, but again our analysis of the environment is so poor we cannot even understand why some do or do not become violent.

similar urban difficulties.[4] Obviously the reason for the difference is contextual. Vancouver does not allow the sale or ownership of handguns, while Seattle does. The same contextual difference likely explains the increasing urban violence elsewhere in the United States. Teenagers and even younger children often get into fights and probably have forever. What differs is the availability of handguns.

I believe it is unfair and untrue to argue that American children in poverty are more aggressive than poor youths in other cultures. How then do we explain the greater murder rate? The choices are two: either there are biological differences between our population and that of other countries, or there is a long-term contextual basis for the difference in murder rates. The test of such a proposition is easy. All that is needed is to alter the contextual variable. In altering the contextual variable, the behavior should alter. From the point of view that I have argued, the altering of behavior will be effective whenever we can alter the context on a long-term basis. If children do not possess an enduring trait, their behavior is contextually determined and maintained. Only the organismic trait model would support the belief that these children are permanently marked by their earlier experience. Quite to the contrary, if their environment is altered, so too is their behavior, as well as the structures that underlie their behavior.

Despite such evidence to the contrary, much of our social policy continues to be driven by the organismic model of development. I have discussed some of the reasons that most social scientists believe the organismic model is correct. An important additional reason is the need to avoid the "blame" for the failure. We prefer to blame violence on individuals rather than looking at the social structure that may support it. So gun manufacturers' and the gun lobby's slogan "Guns don't kill people; people kill people" is quite effective. Of course, that statement is superficially correct, but at its heart it is wrong. Guns do kill people, and without them people have much more difficulty killing other people. Moreover, blaming the victim is now endemic in our American culture. Doctors blame the disease on the patient, lawyers blame the difficulty of the case, teachers blame students for not learning, and therapists blame the clients for not getting better: rarely is it the professionals and their practices who are responsible.

The wish to be relieved of blame is related to unwillingness to institute necessary social reforms. These reforms would be very costly, and this society is not prepared to invest, as, for example, were the Swedes, in making the care of children a top priority.[*] It seems cheaper to try to alter the behavior of specific individuals than to change the structure of the social environment. We are usually more willing to spend large sums of money on studying the genetic and biological causes of aggression than on studying the contextual causes because we hope that the former will lead us to a cure—a onetime versus ongoing expense. And perhaps even more important is the false belief that it is more expensive to alter the environment than cure the person. This unwillingness to pay the piper for the potential causes of social disorganization can be seen almost everywhere. The per-capita expenditure for mildly and profoundly handicapped children is higher than that for poor students in inner-city schools. Society is prepared to spend some money, but not a great deal.

Initiating change in any culture always is associated with the question of cost, and American society seems to have decided that altering the environment is not cost effective. But we have yet to conduct a sufficient test of the idea that with increased resources it is possible to affect, for example, young children's intellectual ability. To test the idea that kids are not biologically stupid (a trait model) but need better environments (a contextual model), both children and family need to be supplied with an array of tutors, special educators, and a set of instructors who spend all of their time working with them. Then, and only then, if they do not learn, is it possible to reject the contextual model and accept the trait model.

As noted earlier, George Bernard Shaw understood the need for contextual change in his play *Pygmalion*, which was made into the popular modern musical *My Fair Lady*. Eliza Doolittle is not given just several hours of instruction, as in the Head Start programs that have been deemed failures; she is brought into Professor Higgins's home. Shaw, of course, was poking fun at the upper-class English when he argued that, by changing her context, he could make Liza into an upper-class Englishwoman. In effect, he was saying that the belief in the trait model was the only way for the upper classes to avoid confronting the reality that people are equal except for contextual differences and that when contextual differences are altered the social differences disappear.

---

[*]In discussing the Swedish experience in reducing childhood injuries, Bergman and Rivara state that "an overriding theme of the campaign initiated in Sweden was that if a nation *valued its children*, their protection had to become a major societal goal" [italics added].[5]

Shaw knew, perhaps better than most developmental psychologists and educators, that the entire context must be changed if a person is to be changed. He also knew that change could come at any point in the life course. Eliza was not changed as a baby; she was a mature adult. That such changes would require enormous resources is an undeniable fact, but before we can say that the cost is *too* high we need to conduct a sufficient, admittedly expensive, test of whether people behave differently when their context changes. Under minimum levels of contextual change, failure to demonstrate the change in children's capacity is likely. This failure allows us to conclude wrongly that the general contextual model, as applied at least to educational opportunity, does not work. Such a conclusion also allows for the restriction of financial resources for such programs.

By and large even the best of those who argue for the more enlightened policies toward children and families are guided by the organismic model. Urie Bronfenbrenner best exemplifies this kind of approach.[6] A noted developmental psychologist, he argues that children's well-being depends on their environments, beginning with the immediate family and extending outward into larger groupings. Bronfenbrenner stresses that the environment at all levels exerts an impact on the family and child and that more than anything else children need people to be "crazy about them." They also need at least two people who will care for them and a policy, governmental as well as industrial, to allow for that. Edward Zigler, a developmental psychologist at Yale University and the first head of the Head Start program in this country, is aligned with Bronfenbrenner in social policy for children. For the last three decades the two have clearly pointed to the importance of context in children's lives, yet their interest in the context of children's lives remains within the framework of the more traditional developmental models: good environments will produce healthy children, and healthy children will make healthy adults. This is a trait model.

I prefer to focus on the underlying models and how they influence social policy. Given the inability to prove the organismic developmental model, I propose that we consider the contextual model. While there is little disagreement between Bronfenbrenner and Zigler and me in terms of the needs of children, I prefer to emphasize contextualism. Perhaps a synthesis of Zigler's and Bronfenbrenner's emphasis on the kind of care children need and the model of contextualism would be best. Following their careful analysis, it is clear that children have special needs: to be cared for by a consistent caregiver, to be loved, to be taught, and to be protected. Supplying these needs during the early part of life is important, but children are not doomed if they do not get them then. Moreover, getting these needs met in early childhood and not thereafter does not protect children from the harm they may encounter later. Children have these needs throughout childhood; we can neither rest if we only supply it early nor fret about the fixity of their fate if they did not receive it at the beginning of their lives.

THE FALLACY OF CAUSE AND EFFECT

Inherent in the trait model is the idea that earlier events in some way affect later ones; in Zigler and Bronfenbrenner's view healthy children will become healthy adults. This leads to the *post hoc, ergo propter hoc* fallacy discussed earlier: if one thing follows another, the first is the cause of the second. True, children crawl before they walk, walk before they talk, and talk before they read; but that these different behaviors are causally related, or even continuous, is impossible to prove. The proposition that development is a closely connected series of events that are linear, causal, and unidirectional cannot be sustained.

Take the belief that abuse leads to abuse. There is widespread support for the idea that intergenerational abuse is related; abused children turn into abusing parents. Cathy Spatz Widom showed that there was little empirical evidence to support the claim of intergenerational abuse. "Among abusing parents, estimates of a history of abuse range from a low of 7% to a high of 70%. Among adults who were abused as children, between one-fifth and one-third abuse their own children."[7] This finding has led Zigler[8] to conclude that the unqualified acceptance of abuse leading to abuse is unfounded.

The fallacy of earlier events causing later ones can also be seen in our views of mental illness. As discussed in Chapter 4, psychologists commonly believe that a child is depressed because the child's depressed mother has imparted some trait to the child, and they usually treat the child by trying to alter that trait or characteristic. But when children are instead removed from the context that produced the characteristic, the trait is likely to disappear, telling us that the child's depression results from the child's being in a depressed environment. If the environment is allowed to continue, it will sustain the behaviors.

What would accepting the contextual model mean for intervention? George goes to a sex therapist because he is suffering from a sexual dysfunction. George can be taught what to do to reduce his problem, and if he has a partner, she too can be taught. In some sense, working with both George and his partner, the sex therapist changes the environment that George is in. Although working with couples has led to considerable success, it is true that the sexually dysfunctional member of the couple must return to an environment in which sexual dysfunction has had a long history. The chance of a significant change in the environment, while possible, is unlikely. Masters, Johnson, Kolodny, and their group, appreciating this predicament, suggested that sexual dysfunctional therapy might be most successful if they could affect not only the individual's behavior but also the environment in which it occurred. They tried to have their patients come to St. Louis and stay in a hotel away from the home environment for several weeks. They also tried surrogate partners. Their experiment suggests an appreciation for the fact that dysfunction, thought to be a property of the individual, is most likely sustained and maintained by the environment, including other people.[9]

THE CRITICAL PERIOD ARGUMENT

Connected with the idea that earlier events affect later ones is the proposition that the earliest events in children's lives have the greatest impact. This is known as the *primacy effect*. Primacy is a powerful variable; the first love of our lives, the first paper published, the first commission made are not forgotten. On the other hand, the *recency effect* is equally powerful; yesterday's meal or movie is more readily recalled than an earlier one. The primacy idea in development often is expressed by the critical period concept. The critical period argument suggests that infancy and early childhood should be emphasized and large resources for intervention during this time committed since this period is more likely to cause changes later. The combination of the critical period concept with the organismic model leads to some unusual beliefs. Perhaps most familiar is the idea Marshall H. Klaus and John H. Kennell developed about "infant bonding." They argued, rather convincingly, that if the child were placed in physical contact with the mother soon after birth, the child and the mother would become bonded to each other and this bonding would lead to adjustment later in life.[10] While the idea of bonding had profound implications for obstetric and postdelivery care, it turns out not to be supported by research.* There was no evidence that it affected subsequent behavior in either infant or mother.

Over ten years ago I was invited to consult with a parent–child program in Philadelphia that involved using a similar bonding interven-tion with teenage inner-city mothers and their children. The interven-tion that these good people tried was the practice of bonding. It was their belief that if they could affect the mother–child relationship during this critical period, they could "inoculate" the mother and child against the adversity that was likely to arise later. Their belief in effecting change later by affecting behavior earlier seems misguided, given the lives these mothers and children were likely to have. The mothers were adolescents, and children themselves. They were uneducated, they had no jobs, and they were likely to live in neighborhoods filled with crime, violence, and drugs. In spite of the fact that mother and child were later to live in horrendous conditions, the model of the critical period allowed the hospital staff to believe that they could affect lives by bonding mother and child in the first half hour after birth. There was no effect of this treatment since the contextual variables that the infant and child lived with overwhelmed any chance that an earlier experience could inoculate them.†

Head Start, the largest of the social intervention programs, is committed to intervening early in children's lives, but if we are informed by a contextual model, other periods of children's lives may be equally important. Not only should Head Start be funded, but additional funds should be created for special programs in middle school and high school, as well as for technical training and adult education. It is only limited funds that force us to choose when to spend our resources. Commitment to a critical period concept re-leases society from its obligation to support educational and other intervention programs across the life span.

---

*Klaus and Kennell required that hospitals introduce lying-in procedures so that mother and child would be in close contact and altered obstetrical practices such that the child, immediately after birth, is given to the mother.[11]

†Parenthetically, it should be pointed out that most reviews of the critical period in literature in human beings are unable to show any effect. Early events, or their lack, do not seem to be critical for later outcomes, most early effects being overridden by current strategies.[12]

MOTHERS AS THE CRITICAL AGENT IN CHILDREN'S DEVELOPMENT

In spite of Bronfenbrenner's ecological approach, and in spite of repeated demonstrations of the significance of others besides the mother, the mother still is treated as the most significant person in the child's environment. Chapter 9 discussed attachment theory, the implications of which for social policy are far-reaching. For example, our beliefs about the mother's role in children's development are complicated by issues of mothers working outside the home and the nature of child care under such circumstances. The issue of the health of children as a consequence of mothers working out of the home and alternative child-care arrangements is a hotly debated topic. Some but not all hold that children will have serious problems in psychosocial adjustment without mothers as their primary caregivers.[13] If we took a contextual view, we might stop worrying about the mother–child relationship and focus on the nature of the environments that children need at each point in their development. All would agree that tender loving care, comfort, and encouragement, as well as protection from harm, are necessary for proper care. Consistent care also is required. Whoever is assigned to care for the child has to remain consistent in the child's life. We can assign a single other or multiple people, but the arrangement must be consistent so as to avoid a chaotic environment where the child does not know who will be caring for him or her. Moreover, the number of children per caregiver must be limited, especially when the children all are of about the same age. Additional factors for proper care include education and perhaps even play. Evidence indicates that men and women of all ages, as well as peers, are needed to satisfy these needs.

The whole issue of whether or not the mother has to be the one to give proper care is very reminiscent of problems that parents in general have with providing care. For example, Suzanne wished for her children to learn to play musical instruments when they were quite young. She did not play a musical instrument. Was it her task to learn how to play and then teach her children, or was it her task to ensure that they got proper instruction? What this example suggests is that it is the parents' task to ensure proper care, not necessarily to give it.

Society is ambivalent as to the role of men in child care, not the least because of Sigmund Freud's idea of the mother as the important person in the child's life. Being a father professionally involved in understanding children's development and involved in caring for my own children, I am rather upset by the relative unimportance the organismic theory accords to fathers. In the human species the presence of an adult male, often the father, is quite important for children's development. That the most accepted theory holds that mothers are the primary force in a child's socioemotional life should offend any male who has loved, cared for, and nurtured his children. Moreover, such a theory, put into practice in the law, often results in fathers losing their rights vis-à-vis their children. But there is a larger issue here. If we rely only on the mother, we neglect all other structures and organizations, as well as people, who can provide care. We need to pay attention to Bronfenbrenner's call for a culture of caring. Structures at all levels of the society are needed to care for and protect our children. I am reminded of having been asked several years ago to help a toy manufacturer produce a game that would teach children about sexual abuse and about being kidnapped. The manufacturer had in mind a game that would teach children how to protect themselves. It struck me as sad that the role of protector and educator had been transferred from adults to the children themselves. Children's need to protect themselves reflects that this society focuses on the mother–child relationship and the within-the-child trait model; because of this emphasis, and the unavailability of mothers, other features of the context of children's lives are ignored.

PROGRESS AND THE IDEA
OF AN END POINT

Early in this book I described the problems that spring from the idea of progress. Progress, implying a series of stages through which one form of functioning gives way to another, more mature level, carries with it the belief in an end point. Both of these ideas impact profoundly on parenting and socialization as well as on more general social policy. The idea of progress, as explained, when applied to socialization practices, leads to the view that the child always is in the process of becoming and never just is. Consequently, parents play with their children to develop children's imagination or creativity in the future[14] rather than because it is fun for the children and enjoyable for them now. Given the argument that it is difficult to demonstrate the antecedents of why children are the way they are now, as well as to predict the consequences of the child's status now for the child's future, there is little reason to suggest to parents or teachers that they should do something for its good effect later. They need to do what they do for children now, not because of their future but because it fits with our current value system. Playing with children is good for them simply because playing is a good thing for children to do. We know it is good because of the current patterns of covariation such as their smiling and attention.

Even though we could not demonstrate, as several studies in the past have been unable to do, that increasing the diet of South American peasant children will lead to increased intellectual performance, there is no reason to believe that we should not feed them. I have been involved in such discussions where the conclusion was reached that because we were unable to demonstrate a positive consequence of altering the nutritional status of poor Colombian children, there was no reason to increase their nutrition. When I pointed out to the assembled scientists that, if this were the case, we should be prepared to reduce the diets of our own children to the level of nutrition that these children have, everyone agreed that this would be a terrible idea. In other words, we should assume, quite independent of the consequences, that eating nutritional meals is good in and of itself.

If we take the idea of progress too seriously, behavior toward children becomes dependent on its consequences rather than on some moral or value system. We feed children, educate children, and care for their health needs because it is better to be fed than to go hungry, better to learn something than to be bored, and better to be healthy than to be ill. These behaviors have face validity because they fit our value system, not because of future consequences for the child.

I always am startled by policy makers' demands that social science demonstrate the effectiveness of current action on subsequent behavior, for example, the need to demonstrate that giving children educational experiences in infancy and early childhood is good for their subsequent school performance. While it certainly would be interesting if such effects could be demonstrated, such a requirement is not made in areas of policy that do not involve social issues. The society spends hundreds of billions of dollars, and has for the last fifty years, on the design, construction, and deployment of atomic and other weapons, under the proposition that this weaponry will safeguard us from war. The expenditure of these resources is justified by the belief that building these weapons will prevent the need to use them. But this hypothesis is never subjected to test since there is no way we could decide whether building these weapons would be a true deterrent. History might provide clues, but our belief in the expenditure of resources is based largely on its face validity, its emotional appeal, and the belief that it will work. Society is willing to expend enormous sums of time, energy, and resources on projects, without the requirement that they work for the future, or at least without any demonstration of it. We increase our police forces in an attempt to limit crime, which does not seem to work. Instead of eliminating such funding, expenditures are increased under the belief that more money is needed. Try doing this for an issue related to children and families!

This society must make a commitment to children and to families not because it will affect the gross national product and not because it necessarily will lead to a better society, although it may well do so, but because it is better to care for children. We should not concern ourselves with the idea of cure. We should concern ourselves with a commitment to caring because it fits within the moral fabric of the society in which we live!

The idea of an end point that accompanies progress may cause even greater problems in social policy. Who determines what the end point is? For Freud the end stage of development occurred once the child solved the Oedipal complex at the age of six years, having passed through the oral, anal, phallic, and genital stages.[15] Erik Erikson, on the other hand, thought about a much larger segment of the life span, which included an end stage in old age.[16] Exploring intellectual development, Jean Piaget saw the final stage of formal operations somewhere in the early adolescent years.[17] In geriatrics the end point is old age. Obviously, there is no absolute end point to development except death.

So it is not surprising that any end point named may be arbitrary. End points are specific to the values and needs of a particular culture at a particular time; end points are relative. Perhaps one of the most celebrated discussions in terms of end point occurred around moral reasoning. Following Piaget, Lawrence Kohlberg argued that moral reasoning followed a sequence, with the end point or highest form of moral reasoning being making decisions based on abstract principles, such as justice, as well as integrating them with the dictates of one's conscience. Kohlberg's research suggested that men showed this type of reasoning more than women. These findings mirrored Freud's earlier belief that women were less moral than men.[18] Carol Gilligan, in her work, argued that the basis for choosing one level as higher than another in regard to moral reasoning was arbitrary.[19] She insisted that the moral reasoning that women were likely to show, reasoning based on caring, personal relationships, and interpersonal obligations, was in no way less mature or less developed than that of men. It was different but not worse. The dispute between Kohlberg and Gilligan should alert us to the danger in believing in some singular end point that represents the goal of some universal progression.

Particular end points of development themselves are a part of the fabric of the sociopolitical beliefs of a system. There may be universals to the process as well as the end point, but the demonstration that this is the case awaits proof, which now is not available. Cultures that differ in values also have different end points. This culture now chooses to believe that the logical, mathematical, scientific thinking that Piaget offered as the end point of intellectual development is reasonable for a culture that is highly technological. However, in cultures in which scientific technology may not exist, such an end point may not be reasonable. A. R. Luria, in the book *Cognitive Development,* argued more for cultural relativism in the type of thinking that characterizes different groups of people.[20] If adaptation to one's environment is a critical feature of successful development, then adaptation to particular cultures with particular cognitive demands should give different end points. Ideas such as that adults are moral and children are amoral, that technological societies are intellectually superior to nontechnological ones, and that the scientific point of view is superior to the religious point of view are part of our value system. The organismic model of development, which demands progress and therefore an end point, leads to the error of equating values with the natural order.

Piaget's theory of genetic epistemology, in which progress occurs as a child moves from practical to abstract knowledge, is a perfect example. The end point of the child's development, and therefore the end point for educational processes, was a structure of thinking that allowed for abstract knowledge. As in the case of moral development, abstract knowledge, or the focus on moral reasoning, was the highest form. But abstract knowledge leads to certain kinds of moral behavior, whereas practical (or social) knowledge leads to others. If the interest is in children's intellectual development, why should the end point be reasoning, rather than how much the person reads or how he uses his intelligence? The choice of end point may be more arbitrary than first considered. For Piaget the end point was a unique kind of reasoning, a reasoning familiar to people in a scientific Western society. Rather than seeing this end point as relative, Piaget chose to make it a universal end point. The commitment to abstract knowledge as the end point of progress results in many schools having curricula that are restricted to this end point. If we reject the idea of progress and end points, it is possible to develop curricula that stress both practical and abstract knowledge.

In my discussion of practical knowledge, I argued that this type of knowledge, something we also call social knowledge, involves the self in knowing. It is knowing through the use of oneself in thinking and feeling. To develop a curriculum for practical or social knowledge, we need to orient our course to the feelings and thoughts of others and to understand others by understanding ourselves. The material of such a curriculum needs to involve topics such as moral behavior, citizenship, and empathy, in addition to trust. All of these topics are based on the idea that how we behave and think about others depends on how we think about ourselves. Remember that in Chapter 7 I said that knowing, which involves abstraction, also involves myself, my experiences, thoughts, and feelings. A curriculum based on practical knowledge has to involve the relation of myself to knowledge of others and my relationship to them. Such knowledge has, as its heart, knowledge about emotions, the feelings of others, and also includes prosocial behavior, which involves such things as empathy and good citizenship, including actions like volunteering to help make a better society.

Before dealing with any of these topics in regard to a curriculum of practical knowledge, we need first to address the question of why we should use our time and energy to focus outside the three R's. Should not reading, writing, and arithmetic be the basis of a school curriculum? At the heart of such an argument is the challenge to ask what the public school's role is in the education of our citizens. If we return to the original motivation for providing public education, we will find that it was predicated on the need not only to educate our diverse immigrant populations into the social fabric of the American way so as to make them good citizens but also to provide them the skills by which they could enter and be successful in our labor force. So even from the beginning of the public education system we understood that its role was to produce good citizens as well as people with the intellectual skills needed for a growing and complex society. From a historical point of view, then, including a practical curriculum is not a radical notion but in fact a return to the original intention of public education.

There is, of course, another argument for a practical and social knowledge curriculum in school. It has been argued by some that part of the social disruption we experience in this latter part of the twentieth century is due to the fact that many of our youngsters cannot read and write and have little arithmetic skill. While this certainly may be true, it neglects the strong possibility that social ills may be due in part to other deficits, including the deficit that I call social or practical knowledge. For example, it is well known that the three leading causes of childhood death are accidents, murders, and suicides. The case might be made that a curriculum based on social or practical knowledge might do more good in altering these distressing statistics than would a curriculum based only on teaching youngsters how to read or write. The social or practical curriculum may produce happier, more well-adjusted children rather than smarter ones. In addition, there is good reason to believe that happier, more well-adjusted children also make better students. Thus, a practical or social knowledge curriculum, rather than acting as a distraction to abstract knowledge, might lead to more productive students and better learning. The net result of omitting such a curriculum is that many students end up learning neither the abstract nor the practical knowledge.

A curriculum of practical and social knowledge should have much to teach. Teaching conflict resolution or respect for others through respect for oneself would be the heart of some of this curriculum. We are familiar with teachers who, in teaching children about the needs and feelings of others with physical and mental handicaps, have the children role-play. In making the child learn by utilizing the self's experience, this role-play results in important understanding. So, for example, children are often asked to go blindfolded for the day to see what a person without sight experiences. This type of curriculum obviously increases the child's understanding of and therefore respect and appreciation for others and their differences.

I am particularly intrigued with the question of volunteering, or behaving in a way so as to be helpful to others by lending one's time, energy, and money. It is clear that no society can survive without this kind of prosocial behavior. In the early-1990s, President George Bush made this the centerpiece of his idea of bettering America when he talked about "a thousand points of light"—the idea that Americans should show good citizenship through volunteering and helping others. Late in 1995, Trenton State College in New Jersey made volunteer work a prerequisite for graduation. This new program is predicated on the idea that the students will learn, through contact with those they help, what it means to help others. Thus the curriculum is designed not only to produce public good but to produce in each student a sense and understanding, a practical knowledge of people who need help and what it feels like to them when they give that help.

Klaus Riegel pointed out that abstract thinking is alienated thinking. It removes from the thought process a self in interaction with the other. Practical knowledge, because it utilizes what we know about ourselves, allows us to treat people as people. People can be empathic because they feel what it is that another knows or feels. When people use abstract knowledge, they cut themselves off from what is known or felt by others. The very abstraction draws them away from people and from their feelings about them.

This kind of thinking occurs in social life all the time. I walk down the street, and a person asks me for some money because he is hungry. I can say, "Gee, I know what it would be like to feel his hunger or the pain of having to beg." By placing myself in his position, my behavior toward him becomes sympathetic and helpful. On the other hand, I can utilize abstract knowledge and remember what percentage of beggars in the street are hungry versus what percentage are more interested in using the money to buy drugs and drink. These abstractions remove me from the practical knowledge of relating to that person.

Whether or not a curriculum of practical knowledge can be devised for school systems remains questionable. However, I have been impressed by a study in which Marilyn Watson, Robert Solomon, and their colleagues have constructed a curriculum around practical moral behavior in the classroom. This curriculum is designed to teach children how to cope in the competitive and noncooperative environment of the classroom, especially how to negotiate needs between students and teacher.[21] The curriculum stresses cooperation and problem solving by making the students think about how their actions affect other students. This type of learning, which utilizes knowledge gained from the self's experiences as taught by the teacher, goes a long way in reducing classroom problems and in increasing such skills as cooperative learning, helping others, and social understanding. To quote from their work:

> It is necessary that one be sensitive to the needs of others before one
> can effectively take those needs into account. Children and adults

vary greatly in their ability to understand the needs and perspectives of others; we therefore include experiences designed to enhance this ability as part of our program.[22]

These kinds of curricula may be important, especially now, in light of the social disorganization manifested in the violence that pervades our schools and streets. Only a model of development that does not stress progress and a single end point can save us from our educational overemphasis on abstraction.

⸻

The nature of development is unclear. The most powerful model our society has utilized, not only to guide research but to order lives, be it in the classroom or in social policy, is the organismic one. A central theme of this model is the idea of progress with a particular end point. It also holds to the ideas of gradualism and continuity of behavior, which allow for the belief that earlier events cause later ones. Such a world view makes us believe we can understand what conditions led to children's and adults' current behavior, and thus we believe we can predict their future behavior.

Within these chapters I have suggested an alternative model of development to help us understand change in light of more recent findings in other fields of science and what they have taught us. As we move to the end of the millennium it seems reasonable to review how the conventional theories of developmental psychology have impacted on our social policy and educational practices and how alternative models could help us solve the enormous social problems facing us in the decades ahead.

The model that I have argued for goes by many names, contextualism being just one. It does not rely on past events as causal explanations for behavior now or require that we predict the future. It is a model that rejects historicism and puts in its stead contextualism and pragmatism as its major principles. How people act currently is determined by their attempt to adapt to situations and problems as they find them. This requires that we focus on the context in which people find themselves and that we observe how they solve the problems that currently exist. Because we cannot predict what will occur in the future, we have only the current to focus on. It means that our caring must be based on our values rather than on what occurred or what will occur. This can be accomplished through a commitment to care for each other now and with an understanding that because we are meaning-seeking creatures, conscious of our existence, we can give up our former quest and accept that unavoidable accidents and chance encounters, discontinuity and chaos, are a part of the nature of human life.

I believe human nature is such that change is always possible. Individuals are always adapting to their environments, and as these environments change, so do people. We change for the good so long as good exists around us. When what is good around us becomes bad, we change again. Without the idea of trait, we are forced to consider the idea of continual adaptation. This means that we must always attempt to create and maintain an environment of good. Creating a good environment for a child at the beginning of life will not have the same effect as an inoculation against mumps.

So the model I propose does not rest on the idea of future gains. It is good for now. What we do now, even if it is good, does not necessarily ensure future good. The fact that it may not necessarily work in the future does not mean it is not worth doing now! Indeed, if it is worth doing now, it should be worth doing in the future as well.

I fear that the idea that doing good for children when they are young is good for their future may not be demonstrated and that critics will continue to use this failure to withhold the time, energy, and resources necessary to do good now.

What is good? It cannot be based on the future but on our sense of what is good *now* for children. What children need is transparent in its simplicity:

- We should be as kind to children as we wish others to be to us.
- We should give children love as we expect to receive it.
- We should excite their senses and stimulate their minds as we wish it for ourselves.
- We should reduce their fears and sadness and increase their interests and joys.
- We should make them care for others as we show them that we care for them.

These needs exist throughout our lives, and it is our job as a just society to give them to our children and to all citizens, not only when they are young but always. Thus each generation passes to the next an ongoing and continuous commitment to maintaining the common good.

Notes

Chapter 1: Chance and Necessity

1. Overton, W. F., & Reese, H. W. (1973). Models of development: Methodological implications. In J. R. Nesselroade & H. W. Reese (Eds.), *Life-span developmental psychology: Methodological issues* (pp. 65–86). New York: Academic Press. Reese, H. W., & Overton, W. F. (1970). Models of development and theories of development. In L. R. Goulet & P. B. Baltes (Eds.), *Life-span developmental psychology: Research and theory* (pp. 115–145). New York: Academic Press.

2. See James, W. (1975). *Pragmatism* (F. Bowers, Text Ed.). Cambridge, MA: Harvard University Press.

3. Schama, S. (1991). *Dead certainties*. London: Granta Books.

4. Taubes, G. (1995). Epidemiology faces its limits. *Science, 269*, 164–169.

5. Jackson, J. B. C., & Cheetham, A. H. (1994). Phylogen reconstruction and the tempo of speciation in cheilostome bryozoa. *Paleobiology, 20,* 407. Kerr, R. A. (1995). Did Darwin get it all right? *Science, 267,* 1421–1422.

6. Rosenbaum, R. (1995). Explaining Hitler. *The New Yorker, 71,* 50–70.

7. Ibid., p. 52.

8. Diamond, J. (1995, January 12). Portrait of the biologist as a young man. *New York Review of Books,* 16.

9. Freud, S. (1950). *The interpretation of dreams* (A. A. Brill, Trans.). New York: Modern Library.

10. Pervin, L. A. (Ed.). (1990). *Handbook of personality: Theory and research*. New York: Guilford Press.

11. Bandura, A. (1982). The psychology of chance encounters and life paths. *American Psychologist, 37,* 747–755.

12. Ross, M. (1989). Relation of implicit theories of the construction of personal histories. *Psychological Review, 96*(2), 341–357.

13. Reese, H. W. (1991). Contextualism and developmental psychology. In

H. W. Reese (Ed.), *Advances in child development and behavior* (Vol. 23, pp. 187–230). New York: Academic Press.

Chapter 2: Three Fixed Ideas

1. Pepper, S. C. (1942). *World Hypotheses*. Berkeley: University of California Press.

2. Mendelson, E. (1980). The continuous and the discrete in the history of science. In O. G. Brim, Jr., & J. Kagan (Eds.), *Constancy and change in human development* (pp. 75–112). Cambridge, MA: Harvard University Press.

3. Merz, J. T. (1914). *A history of European thought in the nineteenth century* (Vol. 4, p. 435). Edinburgh: W. Blackwood & Sons.

4. Bornstein, M., & Krasnegor, N. A. (Eds.). (1989). *Stability and continuity in mental development: Behavioral and biological perspectives*. Hillsdale, NJ: Erlbaum. Brim, O. G., & Kagan, J. (Eds.). (1980). *Constancy and change in human development*. Cambridge, MA: Harvard University Press. Emde, R. N., & Harmon, R. J. (Eds.). (1984). *Continuities and discontinuities in development*. New York: Plenum.

5. Skinner, B. F. (1948). *Walden Two*. New York: Macmillan.

6. Stone, L. (1977). *The family, sex, and marriage in England, 1500–1800*. New York: Harper & Row.

7. Miller, A. (1990). *For your own good: Hidden cruelty in child-rearing and the roots of violence* (H. & H. Hannum, Trans.) (p. 21). New York: Noonday Press.

8. Ibid.

9. See also Schneirla, T. C. (1957). The concept of development in comparative psychology. In D. B. Harris (Ed.), *The concept of development* (pp. 78–108). Minneapolis: University of Minnesota Press. Lerner, R. M., & Busch-Rossnagel, N. A. (Eds.) (1981). *Individuals as producers of their development: A life-span perspective*. San Diego: Academic Press.

10. Schama, S. (1991). *Dead certainties*. London: Granta Books.

11. Tuchman, B. W. (1978). *A distant mirror: The calamitous 14th century*. New York: Knopf.

12. See, for example, Elder, G. H., Jr., Modell, J., & Parke, R. D. (Eds.). (1993). *Children in place and time: Developmental and historical insights*. New York: Cambridge University Press.

13. Bowlby, J. (1988). *A secure base: Parent–child attachment and healthy human development*. New York: Basic Books. Main, M., Kaplan, N., & Cassidy, J. (1985). Security in infancy, childhood, and adulthood: A move to the level of representation. *Monographs of the Society for Research in Child Development*, 50(1–2), 66–104. Shaver, P. R., & Hazan, C. (1993). Adult romantic attachment: Theory and evidence. In W. H. Jones & D. Perlman (Eds.), *Advances in personal relationships* (Vol. 4, pp. 29–70). London: Jessica Kingsley.

14. Riegel, K. F. (1979). *Foundations of dialectical psychology* (p. 124). New York: Academic Press.

15. See Lerner, R. M. (1970). *Final solutions: Biology, prejudice, and genocide*. University Park: Pennsylvania State University Press.

16. Kuhn, T. S. (1970). *The structure of scientific revolutions*. Chicago: University of Chicago Press. Popper, K. R. (1963). *Conjectures and refutations: The growth of scientific knowledge*. London: Routledge & Kegan Paul.

Chapter 3: Traditional Models of Change

1. Pervin, L. A. (Ed.). (1990). *Handbook of personality: Theory and research*. New York: Guilford Press.

2. Jung, C. (1963). *Psychology of the unconscious: A study of the transformations and symbolisms of the libido* (B. M. Hinkle, Trans.). New York: Dodd-Mead (original work published 1916). Plomin, R. (1983). Childhood temperament. In B. Lahey & A. Kazdin (Eds.), *Advances in clinical child psychology* (Vol. 6, pp. 45–92). New York: Plenum.

3. Allport, G. W. (1937). *Personality: A psychological interpretation* (p. 117). New York: Holt, Rinehart & Winston.

4. Greenberg, J. R., & Mitchell, S. A. (1983). *Object relations in psychoanalytic theory*. Cambridge, MA: Harvard University Press.

5. Erikson, E. (1950). *Childhood and society*. New York: Norton.

6. Lewis, M., & Lee-Painter, S. (1974). An interactional approach to the mother–infant dyad. In M. Lewis & L. A. Rosenblum (Eds.), *The effect of the infant on the caregiver: The origins of behavior* (Vol. 1, pp. 21–48). New York: Wiley. Lewis, M., & Rosenblum, L. A. (Eds.) (1977). *Interaction, conversation, and the development of language* (Vol. 5). New York: Wiley. Pervin, L. A., & Lewis, M. (Eds.). (1978). *Perspectives in interactional psychology*. New York: Plenum.

7. Masters, W. H., Johnson, V. E., & Kolodny, R. C. (Eds.). (1977). *Ethical issues in sex therapy and research*. Boston: Little, Brown.

8. Hoffman, H. S. (1974). Fear mediated processes in the context of imprinting. In M. Lewis & L. A. Rosenblum (Eds.), *The origins of fear* (Vol. 2, pp. 25–48). New York: Wiley.

9. Bornstein, M. (Ed.). (1987). *Sensitive periods in development: Interdisciplinary perspectives*. Hillsdale, NJ: Erlbaum. Lamb, M. E., & Hwang, C. (1982). Maternal attachment and mother-neonate bonding: A critical review. In M. E. Lamb & A. L. Brown (Eds.), *Advances in developmental psychology* (Vol. 2, pp. 1–39). Hillsdale, NJ: Erlbaum.

10. Hoffman (1974), op. cit.

11. Largo, R., von Siebenthal, K., & Wolfensberger, U. (in prep.). Profound

change in toilet training: Does it affect development of bowel and bladder control?

12. Bornstein (1987), op. cit. Lamb & Hwang (1982), op. cit.

13. Everett, S. (1941). Lines written for a school declamation. In *The Oxford dictionary of quotations*. London: Oxford University Press.

14. Wordsworth, W. (1973). My heart leaps up. In H. Bloom & L. Trilling (Eds.), *Romantic poetry and prose: The Oxford anthology of English literature*. New York: Oxford University Press.

15. Mendelson, E. (1980). The continuous and the discrete in the history of science (p. 81). In O. G. Brim, Jr., & J. Kagan (Eds.), *Constancy and change in human development* (pp. 75–112). Cambridge, MA: Harvard University Press.

16. Reese, H. W., & Overton, W. F. (1970). Models of development and theories of development. In L. R. Goulet & P. B. Baltes (Eds.), *Life-span developmental psychology: Research and theory* (p. 141). New York: Academic Press.

17. Alvarez, L. W. (1982). Experimental evidence that an asteroid impact led to the extinction of many species 65 million years ago. *Proceedings of the National Academy of Science, 80*, 627–642. Eldredge, N., & Gould, S. J. (1972). Punctuated equilibria: An alternative to phyletic gradualism. In T. J. M. Schopf (Ed.), *Models in paleobiology* (pp. 82–115). San Francisco: Freeman, Cooper.

18. Kagan, J. (1980). Perspectives on continuity (p. 64). In O. G. Brim, Jr., & J. Kagan (Eds.), *Constancy and change in human development* (pp. 26–74). Cambridge, MA: Harvard University Press.

19. Chomsky, N. (1965). *Aspects of a theory of syntax*. Cambridge, MA: MIT Press.

20. Piaget, J. (1952). *The origins of intelligence in children*. New York: International Universities Press.

21. Freud, S. (1953). Three essays on the theory of sexuality. In J. Strachey (Ed. & Trans.), *The standard edition of the complete psychological works of Sigmund Freud* (Vol. 7, pp. 123–243). London: Hogarth Press (original work published 1905).

22. Bowlby, J. (1988). *A secure base: Parent–child attachment and healthy human development*. New York: Basic Books. Although they make the claim for a transformational model, it is, in fact, not. It is a trait model and therefore continuous.

23. Piaget (1952), op. cit.

24. Bower, T. G. R. (1977). *The perceptual world of the child*. Cambridge, MA: Harvard University Press.

25. Flanagan, O. (1991). *The science of the mind* (pp. 135, 139). Cambridge, MA: Bradford, MIT Press.

26. Pascual-Leone, J. (1990). Intension, intention, and early precursors of will: Constructive epistemological remarks on Lewis' research paradigm. *Psychological Inquiry, 1*(3), 258–260. Sugarman, S. (1987). *Piaget's construction of the child's reality*. Cambridge, England: Cambridge University Press.

27. Mounoud, P. (1990). Consciousness as a necessary transitional phenomenon in cognitive development. *Psychological Inquiry, 1*(3), 253–258.

28. Luria, A. R. (1976). *Cognitive development: Its cultural and social foundations* (M. Cole, Ed.). Cambridge, MA: Harvard University Press.

29. LeDoux, J. (1990). Cognitive and emotional interactions in the brain. *Cognition and Emotions, 3,* 265–289. Pribram, K. H. (1984). Emotion: A neurobehavioral analysis. In K. R. Scherer & P. Ekman (Eds.), *Approaches to emotion* (pp. 13–38). Hillsdale, NJ: Erlbaum.

30. Lyons, J. (1970). *Noam Chomsky.* New York: Viking Press. Gottlieb's book (Gottlieb, G. [1992]. *Individual development and evolution.* New York: Oxford University Press.) suggests that environments can exert considerable effects, for example, may be able to produce language in the higher apes and some environmental factors can prevent language development in children.

31. Lewis, M. (1990). Social knowledge and social development. *Merrill–Palmer Quarterly, 36*(1), 93–116. Lewis, M., & Brooks-Gunn, J. (1979). *Social cognition and the acquisition of self.* New York: Plenum.

32. Lerner, R. M. (1992). *Final solutions: Biology, prejudice, and genocide.* University Park: Pennsylvania State University Press. Lerner, R. M., & von Eye, A. (1992). Sociobiology and human development: Arguments and evidence. *Human Development, 35,* 12–33.

33. Broman, S. H., Nichols, P. L., & Kennedy, W. A. (1975). *Preschool IQ: Prenatal and early development correlates.* Hillsdale, NJ: Erlbaum.

34. Szasz, T. S. (1961). *The myth of mental illness.* New York: Harper.

35. Witkin, H. A., Mednick, S. A., Schulsinger, F., Bakkestrom, E., Christiansen, K. O., Goodenough, D. R., Hirschorn, K., Lundsteen, C., Owen, D. R., Philip, J., Rubin, D. B., & Stocking, M. (1976). Criminality in XYY and XXY men. *Science, 193,* 547–555.

36. Wilson, E. O. (1975). *Sociobiology.* Cambridge, MA: Belknap Press of Harvard University.

37. Mounoud, P. (1976). Les révolutions psychologiques de l'enfant [Psychological revolutions during childhood]. *Archives de Psychologie, 44,* 103–114.

38. Wilson (1975), op. cit.

39. Plomin, R. (1990). *Nature and nurture.* Pacific Grove, CA: Brooks/Cole.

Chapter 4: Development in Context

1. James, W. (1950). *Principles of psychology.* New York: Dover (original work published 1890 by Holt). James, W. (1975). *Pragmatism* (F. Bowers, Text Ed.). Cambridge, MA: Harvard University Press.

2. Pepper, S. C. (1942). *World hypotheses.* Berkeley: University of California Press.

3. James (1950), op. cit., Vol. 1, p. 462.

4. See, for example, Ford, D. H., & Lerner, R. M. (1992). *Developmental systems theory: An integrative approach*. Newbury Park, CA: Sage.

5. Pepper (1942), op. cit., p. 240.

6. Bruner, J. (1990). *Acts of meaning* (p. 21). Cambridge, MA: Harvard University Press.

7. Gergen, K. J. (1973). Social psychology as history. *Journal of Personality and Social Psychology, 26*, 309–320. Gergen, K. J. (1980). The emerging crisis in life-span developmental theory. *Life-Span Development and Behavior, 3*, 31–63.

8. Kierkegaard, S. (1846). *The present age* (A. Duc, Trans.). New York: Harper & Row.

9. Morgan, C. L. (1961). C. Lloyd Morgan. In C. Murchison (Ed.), *A history of psychology in autobiography* (Vol. 2, pp. 237–264). New York: Russell & Russell (original work published 1932).

10. Ross, M. (1989). Relation of implicit theories of the construction of personal histories. *Psychological Review, 96*(2), 341–357.

11. Ibid., p. 342.

12. Ibid., p. 346.

13. Reiter, H. L. (1980). The perils of partisan recall. *Public Opinion Quarterly, 44*, 385–388.

14. Collins, L. M., Graham, J. W., Hansen, W. B., & Johnson, C. A. (1985). Agreement between retrospective accounts of substance use and earlier reported substance use. *Applied Psychological Measurement, 9*, 301–309.

15. Yarrow, M. R., Campbell, J. D., & Burton, R. V. (1970). Recollections of childhood: A study of the retrospective method. *Monographs of the Society for Research in Child Development, 35*(5).

16. Ibid., p. 41.

17. Ibid., p. 48.

18. Bowlby, J. (1980). *Attachment and loss: Loss, sadness, and depression*. New York: Basic Books. See also Bretherton, I. (1990). Open communication and internal working models: Their role in the development of attachment relationships. In R. A. Thompson (Ed.), *Nebraska symposium on motivation: Socioemotional development* (pp. 57–113). Lincoln: University of Nebraska Press.

19. Rovee-Collier, C., Early, L., & Stafford, S. (1989). Ontogeny of early event memory: III. Attentional determinants of retrieval at 2 and 3 months. *Infant Behavior and Development, 12*(2), 147–161.

20. Goodman, G. S., & Clarke-Stewart, A. (1991). Suggestibility in children's testimony: Implications for sexual abuse investigations. In J. Doris (Ed.), *The suggestibility of children's recollections: Implications for eyewitness testimony* (pp. 92–105). Washington, DC: American Psychological Association.

21. Kahneman, D., & Snell, J. (1992). Predicting a changing taste. *Journal of Behavioral Decision Making, 5*, 187–200.

22. Nozick, N. (1981). *Philosophical explanation*. Cambridge, MA: Beklap Press at Harvard University.

23. Lewis, M., & Feiring. C. (1991). Attachment as personal characteristic or a measure of the environment. In J. L. Gewirtz & W. M. Kurtines (Eds.), *Intersections with attachment* (pp. 3–22). Hillsdale, NJ: Erlbaum.

24. Elder, G. H., Jr. (1986). Military times and turning points in men's lives. *Developmental Psychology, 22*, 233–245.

25. Bandura, A. (1982). The psychology of chance encounters and life paths. *American Psychologist, 37*, 747–755.

26. Whitehead, A. N. (1978). *Process and reality: An essay in cosmology* (p. 233). New York: Free Press (original work published 1929).

Chapter 5: Progress and the Metaphor of Development

1. Ford, D. H., & Lerner, R. M. (1992). *Developmental systems theory: An integrative approach*. Newbury Park, CA: Sage.

2. Lasch, C. (1991). *The true and only heaven: Progress and its critics* (p. 60). New York: Norton.

3. Job 38:2,4,12,17; 39:27; 40:2.

4. Seligman, M. E. P. (1991). *Learned optimism*. New York: Knopf.

5. Lasch (1991), op. cit., p. 61.

6. Ibid., p. 82.

7. Baldwin, J. M. (1894). *Handbook of psychology: Feeling and will*. New York: Holt.

8. Gilligan, C. (1982). *In a different voice*. Cambridge, MA: Harvard University Press.

9. Luria, A. R. (1976). *Cognitive development: Its cultural and social foundations* (M. Cole, Ed.). Cambridge, MA: Harvard University Press.

10. Waldrop, W. M. (1992). *Complexity: The emerging science at the edge of order and chaos*. New York: Touchstone Press.

Chapter 6: Behavior Serves Many Masters

1. Tannen, D. (1992). *You just don't understand: Women and men in conversation*. New York: Morrow.

2. Lewis, M. (1967). The meaning of a response, or why researchers in infant behavior should be oriental metaphysicians. *Merrill–Palmer Quarterly, 13*(1), 7–18.

3. Nesselroade, J. R. (1983). Temporal selection and factor invariance in the study of development and change. In P. B. Baltes & O. G. Brim, Jr. (Eds.), *Life-span development and behavior* (Vol. 5, pp. 59–87). New York: Academic Press. Nesselroade, J. R. (1988). Some implications of the trait–state distinction for the

study of development over the life-span: The case of personality. In P. B. Baltes, D. L. Featherman, & R. M. Lerner (Eds.), *Life-span development and behavior* (Vol. 8, pp. 163–189). New York: Academic Press.

4. Shweder, R. A. (1990). Cultural psychology—What is it? In J. W. Stigler, R. A. Shweder, & G. Herdt (Eds.), *Cultural psychology: Essays on comparative human development* (pp. 1–43). Cambridge, England: Cambridge University Press.

5. Lewis, M. (1993). The development of deception. In M. Lewis & C. Saarni (Eds.), *Lying and deception in everyday life* (pp. 90–105). New York: Guilford Press.

6. Bell, R. Q., Weller, G. M., & Waldrop, M. (1971). Newborn and preschooler: Organization of behavior and relations between periods. *Monographs of the Society for Research in Child Development, 36*(1–2). Kagan, J. (1980). Perspectives on continuity. In O. G. Brim, Jr., & J. Kagan (Eds.), *Constancy and change in human development* (pp. 26–74). Cambridge, MA: Harvard University Press.

7. Lewis, M., & Sullivan, M. W. *Development of anger.* Unpublished manuscript.

8. Ekman, P., & Friesen, W. V. (1975). *Unmasking the face.* Englewood Cliffs, NJ: Prentice-Hall. Izard, C. (1977). *Human emotions.* New York: Plenum. Tomkins, S. S. (1962). *Affect, imagery, consciousness: Vol. 1. The positive affects.* New York: Springer. Tomkins, S. S. (1963). *Affect, imagery, consciousness: Vol. 2. The negative affects.* New York: Springer.

9. Lewis, M., & Michalson, L. (1983). *Children's emotions and moods: Developmental theory and measurement.* New York: Plenum.

10. Lewis (1993), op. cit.

11. Lewis, M. (1992). *Shame: The exposed self.* New York: Free Press.

12. Lewis, M. (1987). Early sex role behavior and school age adjustment. In J. M. Reinisch, L. A. Rosenblum, & S. A. Sanders (Eds.), *Masculinity/femininity: Basic perspectives* (pp. 202–226). New York: Oxford University Press.

13. Green, R. (1974). *Sexual identity conflict in children and adults.* New York: Basic Books.

14. Lerner, R. M. (1984). *On the nature of human plasticity.* New York: Cambridge University Press.

15. Emmerich, W. (1964). Continuity and stability in early social development. *Child Development, 35,* 311–332. Emmerich, W. (1968). Personality development and concepts of structure. *Child Development, 39,* 671–690.

16. This, too, may be an artifact of measurement. See the debates on this subject: Costa, P. T., Jr., & McCrae, R. R. (1980). Still stable after all these years: Personality as a key to some issues in adulthood and old age. In P. B. Baltes & O. G. Brim, Jr. (Eds.), *Life-span development and behavior* (Vol. 3, pp. 65–102). New York: Academic Press. Nesselroade (1983), op. cit. Nesselroade (1988), op. cit. Nesselroade, J. R., Schaie, K. W., & Baltes, P. B. (1972). Ontogenetic and

generational components of structural and quantitative change in adult behavior. *Journal of Gerontology, 27,* 222–228. Horn, J. L., & Donaldson, G. (1977). Faith is not enough: A response to the Baltes–Schaie claim that intelligence does not wane. *American Psychologist, 32*(5), 369–373.

17. Lewis, M., & Brooks, J. (1974). *Self, others and fear: Infants' reactions to people.* Presented at a Conference on the Origins of Behavior: Fear. Princeton, NJ, October 1973; published in M. Lewis & L. Rosenblum (Eds.), *The origins of fear* (Vol. 2, pp. 195–227). New York: Wiley.

18. Barker, R. G. (1965). Explorations in ecological psychology. *American Psychologist, 20,* 1–14.

19. Pervin, L. A. (1975). Definitions, measurements, and classifications of stimuli, situations, and environments. *Research Bulletin, 75–23.* Princeton, NJ: Educational Testing Service.

20. Hayne Reese, personal communication, 1994.

Chapter 7: Newton, Einstein, Piaget, and the Self

1. Lewin, K. (1935). *A dynamic theory of personality: Selected papers by Kurt Lewin* (D. K. Adams & K. E. Zener, Trans.). New York: McGraw-Hill.

2. Pagels, E. (1979). *The gnostic gospels.* New York: Random House.

3. Ibid., p. 226.

4. Hudson, L. (1972). *The cult of the fact.* London: Cape.

5. Ibid. Roe, A. (1951). A psychological study of eminent physical scientists. *General Psychology Monographs, 43,* 121–135. Roe, A. (1953). *The making of a scientist.* New York: Dodd, Mead. Roe, A. (1961). The psychology of the scientist. *Science, 134,* 456–459.

6. Durant, W. (1954). *The story of philosophy* (p. 121). New York: Pocket Books.

7. Ibid., p. 129.

8. Ibid., p. 131.

9. Ibid.

10. Newton, I. (1960). *Mathematical principles of natural philosophy* (p. 6). Berkeley: University of California Press.

11. Schilpp, P. A. (1949). *Albert Einstein: Philosopher-scientist* (p. 19). Evanston, IL: Library of Living Philosophers.

12. Clark, R. W. (1972). *Einstein: The life and times* (p. 182). New York: Avon.

13. Freundlich, E. (1920). *The foundations of Einstein's theory of gravitation* (p. viii). Cambridge, England: Cambridge University Press.

14. Zukav, G. (1979). *The dancing Wu Li masters* (p. 54). New York: Morrow.

15. Bohr, N. (1958). *Atomic physics and human knowledge* (pp. 96–97). New York: Wiley.

16. Zukav (1979), op. cit., p. 118.

17. Judson, H. F. (1980). *The eighth day of creation: Makers of the revolution in biology* (p. 178). New York: Simon & Schuster.

18. Durant (1954), op. cit., p. 131.

19. Maccoby, E. E., & Jacklin, C. N. (1974). *The psychology of sex differences*. Stanford, CA: Stanford University Press.

20. Bohr (1958), op. cit., p. 416.

21. Piaget, J. (1960). *The psychology of intelligence*. New York: Littlefield, Adams. Polyani, M. (1958). *Personal language: Toward a post-critical philosophy*. London: Routledge & Kegan Paul.

22. Bower, G. H., & Gilligan, S. G. (1979). Remembering information related to oneself. *Journal of Research on Personality, 113,* 404–419.

23. Hyde, T. S., & Jenkins, J. J. (1969). The differential effects of incidental tasks on the organization of recall of a list of highly associated words. *Journal of Experimental Psychology, 82,* 472–481. Kuiper, N. A., & Rogers, T. B. (1979). Encoding of personal information: Self-other differences. *Journal of Personality and Social Psychology, 37*(4), 499–514. Rogers, T. B., Kuiper, N. A., & Kirker, W. S. (1977). Self-reference and the encoding of personal information. *Journal of Personality and Social Psychology, 35,* 677–688.

24. Janellen Huttenlocker, personal communication, 1980.

25. Tagiuri, R. (1969). Person perception. In G. Lands & E. Ironstone (Eds.), *The handbook of social psychology: Vol. 3. The individual in a social context* (pp. 395–449). Reading, MA: Addison-Wesley.

26. Asch, S. E. (1952). *Social psychology* (p. 142). Englewood Cliffs, NJ: Prentice Hall.

27. Merleau-Ponty, M. (1964). *The primacy of perception* (J. Eddie, Ed.; W. Cobb, Trans.) (p. 113). Evanston, IL: Northwestern University Press.

28. Bannister, R., & Agnew, J. (1977). The child's construing of self. In A. W. Landfield (Ed.), *Nebraska symposium on motivation* (Vol. 24, pp. 99–125). Lincoln: University of Nebraska Press.

29. Luria, A. R. (1976). *Cognitive development: Its cultural and social foundations* (M. Cole, Ed.). Cambridge, MA: Harvard University Press.

30. Feldman, N. S. (1979). *Children's impressions of their peers: Motivational factors and the use of inference*. Unpublished doctoral dissertation, Princeton University, Princeton, NJ.

31. Feldman (1979), op. cit., pp. 44, 49.

32. Heider, F. (1958). *The psychology of interpersonal relations* (p. 33). New York: Wiley.

33. Kohut, H. (1971). *The analysis of the self*. New York: International Universities Press.

34. Eisenberg, N., & Lennon, R. (1983). Sex differences in empathy and related capacities. *Psychological Bulletin, 94,* 100–131.

35. Gratch, G. (1979). The development of thought and language in infancy. In J. Osofsky (Ed.), *Handbook of infant development* (pp. 457). New York: Wiley.

36. Tulving, E. (1985). How many memory systems are there? *American Psychologist, 40,* 385–398.

37. Gergen, K. J. (1991). *The saturated self: Dilemmas of identity in contemporary life* (p. 133). New York: Basic Books.

Chapter 8: Consciousness and Being

1. Pervin, L. A. (Ed.). (1990). *Handbook of personality: Theory and research.* New York: Guilford Press.

2. Mischel, T. (1976). Psychological explanations and their vicissitudes. In W. J. Arnold (Ed.), *Nebraska symposium on motivation* (Vol. 23, p. 180). Lincoln: University of Nebraska Press.

3. Boring, E. G. (1950). *A history of experimental psychology.* New York: Appleton.

4. Sartre, J.-P. (1956). *Being and nothingness: An essay on phenomenological ontology* (H. F. Barnes, Trans.). New York: Philosophical Library.

5. Searle, J. R. (1990). Consciousness, explanatory inversion, and cognitive science. *Behaviorial and Brain Sciences, 13,* 586.

6. Freud, S. (1959). Some psychological consequences of the anatomical distinction between the sexes. In J. Strachey (Ed. & Trans.), *The standard edition of the complete psychological works of Sigmund Freud* (Vol. 19, pp. 241–258). London: Hogarth Press (original work published 1925).

7. Stuss, D. T. (1991). Self, awareness, and the frontal lobes: A neuro-psychological perspective. In J. Strauss & G.R. Goethals (Eds.), *The self: Interdisciplinary approaches* (pp. 255–278). New York.

8. Lewis, M. (1992). *Shame: The exposed self.* New York: Free Press.

9. Csikszentmihalyi, M. (1990). *Flow: The psychology of optimal experience.* New York: HarperCollins.

10. Pribram, K. H. (1984). Emotion: A neurobehavioral analysis. In K. R. Scherer & P. Ekman (Eds.), *Approaches to emotion* (pp. 13–38). Hillsdale, NJ: Erlbaum.

11. Bechara, A., Tranel, D., Damasio, H., Adolphs, R., Rockland, C., & Damasio, A. R. (1995). Double dissociation of conditioning and declarative knowledge relative to the amygdala and hippocampus in humans. *Science, 269,* 1115–1118.

12. Gallup, G. G., Jr. (1977). Self-recognition in primates: A comparative approach to the bidirectional properties of consciousness. *American Psychologist, 32,* 329–338.

13. Bechara et al. (1995), op. cit.

14. Pribram (1984), op. cit., p. 111.

15. Babinski, J. (1914). Contribution à l'étude des troubles mentaux dans l'hémiplégie organique cérébrale (anosognosie). *Revue Neurologique, 27,* 845–848. Sacks, O. (1985). *The man who mistook his wife for a hat.* New York: Summit Books.

16. Weiskrantz, L. (1986). *Blindsight: A case study and implications.* New York: Oxford University.

17. Gazzaniga, M. S. (1985). *The social brain: Discovering the networks of the mind.* New York: Basic Books.

18. Emde, R. N. (1983). The prerepresentational self and its affective core. *Psychoanalytic Study of the Child, 38,* 165–192. Freud, S. (1963). *The problem of anxiety* (H.A. Bunker, Trans.) (p. 80). *Object relations theory and clinical psychoanalysis.* New York: Aronson. Kernberg, O. F. (1980). *Internal world and external reality: Object relations theory applied.* New York: Aronson. Lacan, J. (1968). *Language of the self.* Baltimore, MD: Johns Hopkins University Press. Rank, O. (1929). *The trauma of birth.* London: Kegan, Paul,Trench, & Trubner. Stern, D. N. (1985). *The interpersonal world of the infant: A review from psychoanalysis and developmental psychology.* New York: Basic Books.

19. Laing, R. D. (1970). *Knots.* New York: Pantheon Books.

20. For a discussion of this problem, see Putnam, H. (1981). *Reason, truth and history.* Cambridge, England: Cambridge University Press.

21. The topic of self-recognition in infants and young children has been covered in detail in Lewis, M., & Brooks-Gunn, J. (1979). *Social cognition and the acquisition of self.* New York: Plenum.

22. Butterworth, G. (1990). Origins of self-perception in infancy. In D. Cicchetti & M. Beeghly (Eds.), *The self in transition: Infancy to childhood* (pp. 119–137). Chicago: University of Chicago Press.

23. Lewis & Brooks-Gunn (1979), op. cit.

24. Lewis (1992), op. cit.

25. Mead, G. H. (1972). *Mind, self, and society.* Chicago: University of Chicago Press (Original work published 1934). Sullivan, H. S. (1953). *The interpersonal theory of psychiatry.* New York: Norton.

26. Hinde, R. A. (1979). *Towards understanding relationships.* London: Academic Press.

27. Emde (1983), op. cit. Emde, R. N. (1988). Development terminable and interminable. II: Recent psychoanalytic theory and therapeutic considerations. *International Journal of Psychoanalysis, 69,* 283–296. See also Meares, R. (1993). *The metaphor of play: Disruption and restoration in the borderline experience.* Northvale, NJ: Aronson.

28. Mahler, M. S., Pine, F., & Bergman, A. (1975). *The psychological birth of the infant.* New York: Basic Books. Main, M., Kaplan, N., & Cassidy, J. (1985).

Security in infancy, childhood, and adulthood: A move to the level of representation. *Monographs of the Society for Research in Child Development, 50*(1–2), 66–104. Bretherton, I. (1987). New perspectives on attachment relations: Security, communication, and internal working models. In J. D. Osofsky (Ed.), *Handbook of infant development* (2nd ed., pp. 1061–1100). New York: Wiley. Bowlby, J. (1973). *Attachment and loss: Vol. 2. Separation* (p. 208). New York: Basic Books.

Chapter 9: Adaptation and the Nature of Social Life

1. Ainsworth, M. D. S., Blehar, M. C., Waters, E., & Walls, S. (1978). *Patterns of attachment: A psychological study of the strange situation.* Hillsdale, NJ: Erlbaum. Bowlby, J. (1969). *Attachment and loss: Vol. 1. Attachment.* New York: Basic Books.

2. For some of the work showing the infant's exquisite adaptive abilities vis-à-vis his social world, see Eimas, P. D., Siqueland, E. R., Jusczyk, P., & Vigorito, H. (1971, January 22). Speech perception in infants. *Science, 171,* 303–306. Molfese, D. L., Freeman, R. B., & Palermo, D. S. (1975). The ontogeny of brain lateralization for speech and non-speech stimuli. *Brain and Language, 2,* 356–368. Papousek, H. (1981). The common in the uncommon children: Comments on the child's integrative capacities and on initiative parenting. In M. Lewis & L. Rosenblum (Eds.), *The uncommon child* (Vol. 3, pp. 317–328). New York: Plenum. Sander, L. W. (1975). Infant and caretaking environment: Investigation and conceptualization of adaptive behavior in a system of increasing complexity. In E. J. Anthony (Ed.), *Explorations in child psychiatry* (pp. 129–166). New York: Plenum. Streeter, L. A. (1975, March). The effects of linguistic experience on phonetic perception. *Dissertation Abstracts International, 35*(9-B), 4696.

3. Bronfenbrenner, U. (1979). *The ecology of development.* Cambridge, MA: Harvard University Press.

4. Howes, C., Rodning, C., Galluzzo, D. C., & Myers, L. (1988). Attachment and child care: Relationships with mother and caregiver. *Early Childhood Research Quarterly, Special Issue: Infant Day Care, 3,* 403–416. Reprinted in N. Fox & G. G. Fein (Eds.), *Infant day care: The current debate* (pp. 169–182). Norwood, NJ: Ablex. Howes, C., & Hamilton, C. E. (1992). Children's relationships with child care teachers: Stability and concordance with parental attachment. *Child Development, 63,* 867–878. Howes, C., & Hamilton, C. E. (1993). The changing experience of child care: Changes in teachers and in teacher–child relationships and children's social competence with peers. *Early Childhood Research Quarterly, 8,* 15–32. Howes, C., Phillipsen, L., & Galinsky, E. (in press). Girls and boys, teachers and peers: Relationships within a child care center. In C. Howes & C. E. Hamilton (Eds.), *Forming relationships: Children in child care.*

5. Passman, R. H. (1976). Arousal reducing properties of attachment objects: Testing the functional limits of the security blanket relative to the mother. *Developmental Psychology, 12*(5), 468–469.

6. Fox, N. A., Kimmerly, N. L., & Schafer, W. D. (1991). Attachment to mother/attachment to father: A meta-analysis. *Child Development, 62*(1), 210–225. Lewis, M., & Schaeffer, S. (1981). Peer behavior and mother-infant interaction in maltreated children. In M. Lewis & L. Rosenblum (Eds.), *The uncommon child* (Vol. 3, pp. 193–223). New York: Plenum.

7. For a more complete review of the studies on the role of others in the child's social world; see Lewis, M. (1987). Social development in infancy and early childhood. In J. D. Osofsky (Ed.), *Handbook of infant development* (2nd ed., pp. 419–493). New York: Wiley; also Lewis, M. (Ed.). (1984). *Beyond the dyad.* New York: Plenum. Lewis, M., & Rosenblum, L. (1979). (Eds.). *The child and its family* (Vol. 2). New York: Plenum.

8. Shaver, P. R., & Hazan, C. (1993). Adult romantic attachment: Theory and evidence. In W. H. Jones & D. Perlman (Eds.), *Advances in personal relationships* (Vol. 4, pp. 29–70). London: Jessica Kingsley.

9. Harlow, H. F., & Harlow, M. K. (1965). The affectional systems. In A. M. Schrier, H. F. Harlow, & F. Stollnitz (Eds.), *Behavior of nonhuman primates* (Vol. 2, pp. 287–334). New York: Academic Press.

10. Ibid. Hartup, W. W. (1987). Peer relations and family relations: Two social worlds. In M. Rutter (Ed.), *Developmental psychiatry* (pp. 280–292). Washington, DC: American Psychiatric Press. Lewis & Schaeffer (1981), op. cit. Lewis, M., Young, G., Brooks, J., & Michalson, L. (1975). The beginning of friendship. In M. Lewis & L. A. Rosenblum (Eds.), *Friendship and peer relations* (Vol. 4, pp. 27–65). New York: Wiley.

11. Lewis & Schaeffer (1981), op. cit.

12. Block, J., & Haan, N. (1971). *Lives through time.* Berkeley, CA: Bancroft Books. Sroufe, L. A. (1979). Socioemotional development. In J. D. Osofsky (Ed.), *Handbook of infant development* (pp. 462–516). New York: Wiley.

13. Thompson, R. A., & Lamb, M. E. (1984). Infants, mothers, families, and strangers. In M. Lewis (Ed.), *Beyond the dyad* (Vol. 4, pp. 195–221). New York: Plenum Press.

14. Ibid.

15. Fantz, R. L. (1964, October 30). Visual experience in infants: Decreased attention to familiar patterns relative to novel ones. *Science, 146*, 668–670. Fantz, R. L., & Miranda, S. B. (1975). Newborn attention to form or contour. *Child Development, 46*(1), 224–228.

16. Lewis, M., & Goldberg, S. (1969). Perceptual–cognitive development in infancy: A generalized expectancy model as a function of the mother–infant interaction. *Merrill–Palmer Quarterly, 15*(1), 81–100.

17. Ainsworth et al. (1978), op. cit. Lewis & Goldberg (1969), op. cit.

18. Bell, S. M., & Ainsworth, M. D. S. (1972). Infant crying and maternal responsiveness. *Child Development, 42,* 1171–1190. Spock, B. (1983). *Baby and Child Care.* New York: Dutton.

19. Gewirtz, J. L., & Boyd, E. F. (1977). Does maternal responding imply reduced infant crying? A critique of the 1972 Bell and Ainsworth report. *Child Development, 48,* 1200–1207.

20. Rebelsky, F., & Hanks, C. (1971). Fathers' verbal interaction with infants in the first three months of life. *Child Development, 43,* 63–68.

21. Harlow, H. F, & Zimmerman, R. R. (1959). Affectional responses in the infant monkey. *Science, 130,* 421–432.

22. Harlow, H. F. (1958). The nature of love. *American Psychologist, 13,* 673–85. Harlow, H. F. (1961). The development of affectional patterns in infant monkeys. In B. M. Foss (Ed.), *Determinants of infant behavior* (pp. 75–97). London: Methuen. Harlow, H. F. (1969). Age-mate or peer affectional system. In D. S. Lehrman, R. A. Hinde, & E. Shaw (Eds.), *Advances in the study of behavior* (Vol. 2, pp. 333–383). New York: Academic Press. Harlow & Harlow (1965), op. cit. Harlow, H. F., & Harlow, M. K. (1969). Effects of various mother–infant relationships on rhesus monkey behaviors. In B. M. Foss (Ed.), *Determinants of infant behavior* (Vol. 4, pp. 15–36). London: Methuen.

23. Rosenblum, L. A. (1961). *The development of social behavior in the rhesus monkey.* Unpublished doctoral dissertation, University of Wisconsin, Madison.

24. Suomi, S. J., & Harlow, H. F. (1972). Social rehabilitation of isolate-reared monkeys. *Developmental Psychology, 6,* 487–496. Suomi, S. J., & Harlow, H. F. (1975). The role and reason of peer relationships in rhesus monkeys. In M. Lewis & L. A. Rosenblum (Eds.), *Friendship and peer relations* (pp. 153–185). New York: Wiley. Suomi, S. J., & Harlow, H. F. (1978). Early experience and social development in rhesus monkeys. In M. E. Lamb (Ed.), *Social and personality development* (pp. 252–271). New York: Holt, Rinehart & Winston.

25. Hunt, J. M. (1961). *Intelligence and experience.* New York: Ronald. Spitz, R. A. (1946). Analytic depression. *Psychoanalytic Study of the Child, 2,* 313–342. Spitz, R. A. (1950). Anxiety in infancy: A study of its manifestations in the first year of life. *International Journal of Psychoanalysis, 31,* 138–143. Spitz, R. A. (1955). A note on the extrapolation of ethological findings. *International Journal of Psychoanalysis, 36,* 162–165. Spitz, R. A. (1957). *No and yes.* New York: International Universities Press.

26. Yarrow, L. J. (1963). Research in dimensions of early maternal care. *Merrill–Palmer Quarterly, 9,* 101–114.

27. Provence, S., & Lipton, R. (1962). *Infants in institutions.* New York: International Universities Press.

28. Cicchetti, D., & Rizley, R. (1981). Developmental perspectives on the etiology, intergenerational transmission, and sequelae of child maltreatment. *New Directions for Child Development, 11,* 31–55.

29. Bronson, G. W. (1972). Infants' reactions to unfamiliar persons and novel objects. *Monographs of the Society for Research in Child Development, 37*(3). Kagan, J. (1971). *Change and continuity in infancy.* New York: Wiley.

30. Brooks, J., & Lewis, M. (1976). Infants' responses to strangers: Midget, adult, and child. *Child Development, 47,* 323–332. Lewis, M., & Rosenblum, L. A. (Eds.). (1974). *The origins of fear.* New York: Wiley. Walsh, P. V., Katz, P. A., & Downey, E. P. (1991, April 17). *A longitudinal perspective on race and gender socialization in infants and toddlers.* Paper presented at the meeting of the Society for Research in Child Development, Seattle, WA.

31. Lewis, M. (1985). Age as a social dimension. In T. Field & N. Fox (Eds.), *Social perception in infants* (pp. 299–319). New York: Academic Press.

32. Lewis (1987), op. cit.

33. Brooks & Lewis (1976), op. cit..

34. Rosenblum, L. A. (1971). Kinship interaction patterns in pigtail and bonnet macaques. In J. Biegert (Ed.), *Proceedings of the Third International Congress of Primatology* (pp. 79–84). Basel: Karger.

35. Robertson, J., & Robertson, H. (1971). Young children in brief separation: A fresh look. *Psychoanalytic Study of the Child, 26,* 264–315.

36. Konner, M. (1975). Relations among infants and juveniles in comparative perspective. In M. Lewis & L. Rosenblum (Eds.), *Friendship and peer relations* (Vol. 4, pp. 99–129). New York: Wiley.

37. Dunn, J. F., & Kendrick, C. (1982). *Siblings: Love, envy and understanding.* London: Grant McIntyre. Lamb, M. (Ed.). (1981). *The role of the father in child development* (2nd ed.) New York: Wiley.

38. Lewis, M., & Feiring. C. (1979). The child's social network: Social object, social functions, and their relationship. In M. Lewis & L. A. Rosenblum (Eds.), *The child and its family* (Vol. 2, pp. 9–27). New York: Plenum Press.

39. Lamb (1981), op. cit. Pederson, F. A. (Ed.). (1980). *The father–infant relationship: Observational studies in the family setting.* New York: Praeger.

40. Fox et al. (1991), op. cit.

41. Dunn & Kendrick (1982), op. cit.

42. Lewis et al. (1975), op. cit.

43. Howes & Hamilton (1992), op. cit. Howes & Hamilton (1993), op. cit. Howes et al. (1988), op. cit. Howes et al. (in press), op. cit. Howes, C., & Segal, J. (1993). Children's relationships with alternative caregivers: The special case of maltreated children removed from their homes. *Journal of Applied Developmental Psychology, 14,* 71–81. Jaeger, E., & Weinraub, M. (1990). Early non-maternal care and infant attachment: In search of process. *New Directions for Child Development, 49,* 71–90.

44. Clarke-Stewart, K. A. (1978). And daddy makes three: The father's impact on mother and young child. *Child Development, 49*(2), 466–478.

45. Rosenblatt, J. (1974). Behavior in public places: Comparisons of couples

accompanied and unaccompanied by children. *Journal of Marriage and the Family*, 36, 750–755.

46. Lewis, M., & Feiring, C. (1982). Some American families at dinner. In L. Laosa & I. Sigel (Eds.), *The family as a learning environment for children* (Vol. 1, pp. 115–145). New York: Plenum.

47. Parke, R. D., Power, T. G., & Gottman, J. M. (1979). Conceptualizing and quantifying influence patterns in the family triad. In M. E. Lamb, S. J. Suomi, & G. R. Stephenson (Eds.), *Social interaction analysis: Methodological issues* (pp. 231–252). Madison: University of Wisconsin Press.

48. Cairns, R. B, & Hood, K. E. (1983). Continuity in social development: A comparative perspective on individual difference prediction. In P. B. Baltes & O. G. Brim, Jr. (Eds.), *Life-span development and behavior* (Vol. 5, pp. 301–358). New York: Academic Press.

49. Dunn, J., & Kendrick, C. (1980). The arrival of a sibling: Changes in interaction between mother and first-born child. *Journal of Child Psychology and Psychiatry*, 21, 119–132. Dunn, J., Kendrick, C., & MacNamee, R. (1981). The reaction of first-born children to the birth of a sibling: Mothers' reports. *Journal of Child Psychology and Psychiatry*, 22, 1–18.

50. Wilson, E. O. (1975). *Sociobiology*. Cambridge, MA: Belknap Press of Harvard University. Murray, H. A. (1938). *Explorations in personality*. New York: Oxford University Press.

Chapter 10: Time, Sudden Change, and Catastrophe

1. Lyell, C. (1833). *Principles of geology* (Vol. 3, p. 18). London: John Murray.

2. Darwin, C. (1871). *On the origin of species* (p. 14). London: John Murray.

3. Lightman, A. (1993). *Einstein's Dreams* (p. 137). New York: Pantheon.

4. Fraisse, P. (1964). *The psychology of time*. London: Eyre & Spottiswoode. Nisbet, R. (1980). *History of the idea of progress*. New York: Basic Books. Riegel, K. F. (1972). Time and change in the development of the individual society. In H. W. Reese (Ed.), *Advances in child development and behavior* (Vol. 7, pp. 81–113). New York: Academic Press. Riegel, K. F. (1977). The dialectics of time. In N. Datan & H. W. Reese (Eds.), *Life-span developmental psychology: Dialectical perspectives on experiment research* (pp. 3–45). New York: Academic Press.

5. Bergson, H. (1913). *Time and free will*. London: George Allen.

6. Damascius, quoted in Ariotti, P. E. (1975). The concept of time in Western antiquity. In J. T. Fraser & N. Lawrence (Eds.), *The study of time II: Proceedings of the second conference of the International Society for the Study of Time, Lake Yamanaka, Japan* (p. 73). Berlin: Springer.

7. Nisbet, R. (1980). *History of the idea of progress*. New York: Basic Books.

8. Ariotti (1975), op. cit..

9. Aristotle (1941). Physics. In R. McKeon (Ed.), *The basic works of Aristotle* (pp. 20–41). New York: Ransom House.

10. Clark, R. W. (1972). *Einstein: The life and times*. New York: Avon.

11. Riegel (1977), op. cit.

12. Fraser, J. T. (1967, February 6). The interdisciplinary study of time. *Annals of the New York Academy of Sciences, 138*(2), 823.

13. Clark (1972), op. cit., p. 117.

14. See Friedman, W. J. (Ed.). (1982). *The developmental psychology of time*. New York: Academic Press. Gergen, K. J., & Gergen, M. M. (1984). Narratives of the self. In T. Sarbin & K. Schube (Eds.), *Studies in social identity* (pp. 254–273). New York: Prager. Reese, H. W., & McCluskey, K. A. (1984). Dimensions of historical constancy and change. In K. A. McCluskey & H. W. Reese (Eds.), *Life-span developmental psychology: Historical and generational effects* (pp. 17–45). Orlando, FL: Academic Press. Riegel (1977), op. cit.

15. Wohlwill, J. F. (1973). *The study of behavioral development*. New York: Academic Press.

16. Lerner, R. M. (1984). *On the nature of human plasticity*. New York: Cambridge University Press.

17. Friedman, W. J. (1982). Conventional time concepts and children's structuring of time. In W. J. Friedman (Ed.), *The developmental psychology of time* (pp. 12–21). New York: Academic Press. Reese & McCluskey (1984), op. cit. Schaie, K. W. (1984). Historical time and cohort effects. In K. A. McCluskey & H. W. Reese (Eds.), *Life-span developmental psychology: Historical and generational effects* (pp. 1–15). Orlando, FL: Academic Press.

18. Feynman, R. P. (1958). Mathematical formulation of the quantum theory of electromagnetic interaction. In J. Schwinger (Ed.), *Selected papers on quantum electrodynamics* (pp. 257–274). New York: Dover.

19. Riegel (1977), op. cit.

20. Carstensen, L. L. (1993). Motivation for social contact across the life span: A theory of socioemotional selectivity. In J. Jacobs (Ed.), *Nebraska symposium on motivation: Vol. 40. Developmental perspectives on motivation* (pp. 250). Lincoln: University of Nebraska Press.

21. Riegel (1977), op. cit. p. 39.

22. Cohler, B. J. (1982). Personal narrative and life course. In P. B. Baltes & O. G. Brim, Jr. (Eds.), *Life-span development and behavior* (Vol. 4, pp. 205–241). New York: Academic Press. Gergen, K. J. (1977). Stability, change and chance in understanding human development. In N. Datan & H. W. Reese (Eds.), *Life-span developmental psychology: Dialectical perspectives on experimental research* (pp. 135–158). New York: Academic Press. Riff, C. D. (1984). Personality development from the inside: The subjective experience of change in adulthood

and agency. In P. B. Baltes & O. G. Brim, Jr. (Eds.), *Life-span development and behavior* (Vol. 6, pp. 243–279). New York: Academic Press.

23. For some recent examples, see Cohler (1982), op. cit. Gergen & Gergen (1984), op. cit. Freeman, M. (1984). History, narrative and life-span developmental knowledge. *Human Development, 27,* 1–19; also Riff (1984), op. cit. For some older examples, see Cottle, T. J. (1976). *Perceiving time.* New York: Wiley; and Fraisse (1964), op. cit.

24. Cohler (1982), op. cit.

25. Riegel (1977), op. cit.

26. See also Lerner, R. M., Skinner, E. A., & Sorell, G. T. (1980). Methodological implications of contextual/dialectic theories of development. In D. F. Hultsch (Chair), Implications of a dialectical perspective for research methodology. *Human Development, 23,* 217–267.

27. Gratch, G. (1979). The development of thought and language in infancy. In J. Osofsky (Ed.), *Handbook of infant development* (pp. 439–461). New York: Wiley. Kagan, J., Keasley, R. B., & Zelazo, P. R. (1978). *Infancy: Its place in human development.* Cambridge, MA: Harvard University Press. Piaget, J. (1952). *The origins of intelligence in children.* New York: International Universities Press.

28. Lewis, M. (1985). Age as a social dimension. In T. Field & N. Fox (Eds.), *Social perception in infants* (pp. 299–319). New York: Academic Press. Lewis, M., & Michalson, L. (1983). *Children's emotions and moods: Developmental theory and measurement.* New York: Plenum Press.

29. Neugarten, B. L., Moore, J. W., & Lowe, J. C. (1965). Age norms, age constraints, and adult socialization. *American Journal of Sociology, 21,* 710–717. Riff (1984), op. cit.

30. For very similar views, see also Datan, N. (1977). After the apple: Post-Newtonian metatheory for jaded psychologists. In M. Datan & H. W. Reese (Eds.), *Life-span developmental psychology: Dialectical perspectives on experimental research* (pp. 47–57). New York: Academic Press; and Sinnott, J. D. (1981). The theory of relativity: A metatheory for development. *Human Development, 24,* 293–311.

31. Eldredge, N., & Gould, S. J. (1972). Punctuated equilibria: An alternative to phyletic gradualism. In T. J. M. Schopf (Ed.), *Models in paleobiology* (pp . 82–115). San Francisco, CA: Freeman, Cooper.

32. Levington, J. S. (1992). The big bang of animal evolution. *Scientific American, 267*(5), 88–89.

33. Gould, S. J. (1980). *The panda's thumb* (p. 181). New York: Norton.

34. Eldredge & Gould (1972), op. cit.

35. University of Chicago paleontologist Jack Sepkoski quoted in Kerr, R. A. (1993, July 16). Even warm climates get the shivers. *Science, 261,* 292.

36. Raup, D. M. (1986, March 28). Biological extinction in earth history. *Science, 231*, 1531–1532.

37. Alvarez, L. W. (1982). Experimental evidence that an asteroid impact led to the extinction of many species 65 million years ago. *Proceedings of the National Academy of Science, 80*, 627–642.

38. Raup (1986), op. cit., p. 1531.

39. Ibid., p. 1532.

40. Lampl, M., Veldhuis, J. D., & Johnson, M. L. (1992, October 30). Saltation and stasis: A model of human growth. *Science, 258*, 801–803.

41. McCall, R. B., Hogarty, P. S., & Hurlburt, N. (1972). Transitions in infant sensorimotor development and the prediction of childhood IQ. *American Psychologist, 27*(8), 728–748.

42. Kerr (1993), op. cit.

43. Feldman, R. O. (1982). *What Ever Happened to the Quiz Kid: Perils and profits of growing up gifted.* Chicago: Chicago Review Press.

44. Diamond, J. (1995, January 13). Portrait of the biologist as a young man. *New York Review of Books*, p. 16.

45. Ibid.

46. Hempel, C. G. (1967). Scientific explanations. In S. Morgenbesser (Ed.), *Philosophy of science today* (pp. 79–88). New York: Basic Books.

47. Gleick, J. (1987). *Chaos, making a new science.* New York: Viking.

48. Thom, R. (1975). *Structural stability and morphogenesis.* Reading, MA: Benjamin. Zeeman, E. C. (1976). Catastrophe theory. *Scientific American, 234*, 65–83.

49. Thelen, E., & Ulrich, B. D. (1991). Hidden skills: A dynamic systems analysis of treadmill stepping during the first year. *Monographs of the Society for Research in Child Development, 56*(1, Serial No. 223). van Geert, P. (1991). A dynamic systems model of cognitive and language growth. *Psychological Review, 98*, 3–53.

50. Poole, R. (1989, February 17). Quantum chaos: Enigma wrapped in a mystery. *Science, 243*, 893–895.

51. Ibid.

52. Lyon, J., & Gorner, P. (1995). *Altered fates: Gene therapy and the retooling of human life.* New York: Norton.

53. See D. L. Pauls (1993). Behavioral disorders: Lessons in linkage. *Nature Genetics, 3*, 4–5. Gora-Maslak, G., McClearn, G. E., Crabbe, J. C., Phillips, T. J., Belknap, J. K., & Plomin, R. (1991). Use of recombinant inbred strains to identify quantitative trait loci in psychopharmacology. *Psychopharmacology, 104*(4), 413–424.

54. Flint, J., Corley, R., DeFries, J. C., Fulker, D. W., Gray, J. A., Miller, S., & Collins, A. C. (1995). A simple genetic basis for a complex psychological trait in laboratory mice. *Science, 269*, 1432–1435.

Chapter 11: Cure or Care

1. Ramey, C. T., & Trohanis, P. L. (Eds.). (1982). *Finding and educating the high-risk and handicapped infants*. Baltimore: University Park Press.

2. Dukes, M. N. G. (1984). Sex hormones. In M. N. G. Dukes (Ed.) & B. Westerholm (Section Ed.), *Meyler's side effects of drugs* (pp. 764–781). New York: Elseviar. Lazar, I., & Darlington, R. B. (1982). Lasting effects of early education: A report from the consortium for longitudinal studies. *Monographs of the Society for Research in Child Development, 47*(2–3, Serial No. 195), 10.

3. Widom, C. S. (1989, April 14). The cycle of violence. *Science, 244*, 163.

4. Sloan, J. H., Kellermann, A. L., Reay, D. T., Ferris, J. A., Koepsell, T., Rivara, F. P., Rice, C., Gray, L., & LoGerfo, J. (1988, November 10). Handgun regulations, crime, assaults, and homicide: A tale of two cities. *New England Journal of Medicine, 319*(19), 1256–1262.

5. Bergman, A. B., & Rivara, F. P. (1991). Sweden's experience in reducing childhood injuries. *Pediatrics, 88*(1), 69–74.

6. Bronfenbrenner, U. (1979). *The ecology of development*. Cambridge, MA: Harvard University Press.

7. Widom (1989), op. cit., p. 160.

8. Kaufman, J., & Zigler, E. (1987). Do abused children become abusive parents? *American Journal of Orthopsychiatry, 57*(2), 186–192.

9. Masters, W. H., Johnson, V. E., & Kolodny, R. C. (Eds.). (1977). *Ethical issues in sex therapy and research*. Boston: Little, Brown.

10. Klaus, M. H., & Kennell, J. H. (1976). *Maternal–infant bonding: The impact of early separation or loss on family development*. St. Louis: Mosby. Klaus, M. H., & Kennell, J. H. (1982). *Parent–infant bonding*. St. Louis: Mosby.

11. Myers, B. J. (1987). Mother–infant bonding as a critical period. In M. H. Bornstein (Ed.), *Sensitive periods in development* (pp. 223–245). Hillsdale, NJ: Erlbaum.

12. Bornstein, M., & Krasnegor, N. A. (Eds.). (1989). *Stability and continuity in mental development: Behavioral and biological perspectives*. Hillsdale, NJ: Erlbaum.

13. Belsky, J. (1988). The "effects" of infant day care reconsidered. *Early Childhood Research Quarterly, Special Issue: Infant Day Care, 3*(3), 235–272. Clarke-Stewart, K. A. (1988). The "effects" of infant day care reconsidered: Risks for parents, children, and researchers. *Early Childhood Research Quarterly, Special Issue: Infant Day Care, 3*(3), 293–318.

14. Singer, D. G., & Singer, J. L. (1977). *Partners in play*. New York: Harper & Row.

15. Freud, S. (1953). Three essays on the theory of sexuality. In J. Strachey (Ed. & Trans.), *The standard edition of the complete psychological works of Sigmund*

Freud (Vol. 7, pp. 123–243). London: Hogarth Press and the Institute of Psychoanalysis (original work published 1905).

16. Erikson, E. (1950). *Childhood and society.* New York: Norton.

17. Piaget, J. (1952). *The origins of intelligence in children.* New York: International Universities Press.

18. Kohlberg, L. (1976). Moral stages and moralization: The cognitive–developmental approach. In T. Lickona (Ed.), *Moral development and behavior: Theory, research, and social issues* (pp. 31–53). New York: Holt, Rinehart & Winston.

19. Gilligan, C. (1982). *In a different voice.* Cambridge, MA: Harvard University Press.

20. Luria, A. R. (1976). *Cognitive development: Its cultural and social foundations* (M. Cole, Ed.). Cambridge, MA: Harvard University Press.

21. Solomon, R., Watson, M., Battistich, V., Schaps, E., & Delucchi, K. (1992). Creating a caring community: Educational practices that promote children's prosocial development. In F. K. Oser, A. Dick, & J. Patry (Eds.), *Effective and responsible teaching: The new synthesis* (pp. 383–396). San Francisco: Jossey-Bass. Watson, M., Solomon, D., Battistich, V., Schaps, E., & Solomon, J. (1989). The child development project: Combining traditional and developmental approaches to values education. In L. P. Nucci (Ed.), *Moral development and character education* (pp. 51–92). Berkeley, CA: McCutchan.

22. Watson et al. (1989), op. cit., p. 59.

INDEX